ACTIVE
SOCIAL WORK WITH
CHILDREN WITH
DISABILITIES

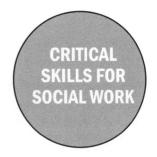

CRITICAL
SKILLS FOR
SOCIAL WORK

ACTIVE
SOCIAL WORK WITH
CHILDREN WITH
DISABILITIES

Julie Adams & Diana Leshone

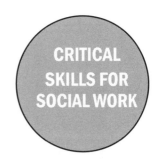

CRITICAL
SKILLS FOR
SOCIAL WORK

First published in 2016 by Critical Publishing Ltd

British Library Cataloguing in Publication Data
A CIP record for this book is available from the British Library

ISBN: 978-1-910391-94-5

This book is also available in the following ebook formats:

MOBI: 978-1-910391-95-2
EPUB: 978-1-910391-96-9
Adobe ebook reader: 978-1-910391-97-6

Cover by Out of House
Text design by Greensplash
Drawing design by Richard Leshone
Project Management by Out of House Publishing
Printed and bound in Great Britain by TJ International, Padstow

Critical Publishing
152 Chester Road
Northwich
CW8 4AL
www.criticalpublishing.com

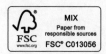

Contents

Help us to help you!

Our aim is to help you to become the best professional you can be. In order to improve your critical thinking skills we are pleased to offer you a **free booklet** on the subject. Just go to our website www.criticalpublishing.com and click the link on the home page. We have more free resources on our website which you may also find useful.

If you'd like to write a review of this book on Amazon, Books Etc, or Wordery, **we would be happy to send you the digital version of the book for free**.

Email a link to your review to us at admin@criticalpublishing.com, and we'll reply with a PDF of the book, which you can read on your phone, tablet or Kindle.

You can also connect with us on:

Twitter @CriticalPub #criticalpublishing

Facebook www.facebook.com/Critical-Publishing-456875584333404

Our blog *https://thecriticalblog.wordpress.com*

Meet the authors

Julie Adams has personal experience of living with a sibling with severe learning disabilities, which led to her starting her social work career in residential care in 1992, working in a respite setting for children with disabilities. After qualifying in 1999 she then moved into field social work, and has worked in a variety of settings, including child protection, adoption and looked-after children. Julie has worked as a team manager in Children with Disability Teams, and also in a hospital setting with adults with complex health needs and learning disabilities. Julie is a qualified practice educator and also delivers training; she co-wrote *Positive Social Work: The Essential Toolkit For NQSWs*.

Diana Leshone began working with children and families in 1989, starting in a Family Centre in partnership with Save the Children and the local authority. Her work includes assessments, direct work with children, crisis response, court work, behaviour management, including developing and delivering courses, parenting skills and disabilities. Diana has managed a Resource Centre and a Children's Centre while continuing to have children's needs in focus. She qualified as a social worker in 2009 and joined a children's disability team, progressing to senior social worker. Diana has delivered training with Julie and is continually looking to share her practice wisdom with others in this field.

Acknowledgements

In writing this book, we would like to acknowledge the following with special thanks:

From Julie to my late, much-treasured mum and brother. My supportive dad and a huge special thank you to my wonderful partner Darren – I love you all.

From Diana to my wonderful, patient and caring family, Alan, James, Richard, Abigail, Dylan and Jayne, my wonderful parents, and not forgetting my grandchildren, Noah and Edith – I love you all.

Introduction

Thank you for choosing *Active Social Work with Children with Disabilities*. We hope this book will help you enhance your learning and understanding, and dispel any fears you may have about entering this most wonderful and rewarding area of social work practice. Our main target audience is those who are working as social workers, particularly students, those who are newly qualified, or social workers who have not worked with children with disabilities before. Throughout the book, and then in one specially dedicated chapter, there are many activities that can be completed by social workers and practice educators with their students on placement, or within supervision and/or team meetings to support with Continued Professional Development (CPD). The exercises are also suitable for those social workers undertaking training on their Assessed and Supported Year in Employment (ASYE) to help evidence their learning and reflective practice on each activity.

Why did we write this book? We wanted to introduce you to some of the different, and often very difficult, aspects of social work practice with children with disabilities that we have experienced and had to overcome along the way. Our approach includes: helping you understand some of the legislation and putting it into straightforward language with illustrative examples; exploring the processes you are working within; and giving you some strategies for managing the emotional impact of disability, which we believe to be one of the most difficult areas of working with children with disabilities and those children with limited life expectancy. We also explore another significant area of importance that is always a challenge and one many fear they cannot do: communicating with children with disabilities. We give tips for undertaking your assessment and give some behaviour management advice and strategies, which we hope you will find useful and help you understand and explore values and ethics, and signpost you to useful resources for families.

This book is designed to gently guide you through the emotional and challenging experiences you will undoubtedly encounter on your journey with real children and their families. You will begin to recognise your own levels of emotional intelligence through reading some case scenarios of real families' situations, which have the aim of helping you understand the sometimes difficult emotional journeys you will take with the families, and more importantly the emotional strength and resilience you will need to find within yourself to cope with your professional experiences.

We want to share some of our experiences as a way of trying to offer you an insight into this specialist area of social work. It is also important to explain here that while we have shared some strategies, approaches and guidance, these are just ideas and practice wisdom, and are by no means the answers or ideal approaches that would suit other situations. As you may have gathered by now social work is very different to other professions in that there is no instruction book or manual to tell you how to manage or approach a situation; it takes a good level of emotional intelligence, mixed with honesty, respect and a true desire to make a positive difference to the families you will work with. It would be great if it was like a mathematical equation as 2+2 will always equal 4, but disability + mental health will never have the same result for everyone.

We understand that it is difficult to achieve fully appropriate terms within the whole book, and would like to stress that if there are any terms used that offend this is not our intention: we have tried to get the terminology right in terms of describing the needs of children with disabilities, recognising the children as people first, and not to get into labelling the child – only the disability. Here, we would also like to give a huge THANK YOU to all the children, young people, families and colleagues who contributed to the book.

We would like to begin this book by including some words of wisdom and experience from a parent who had taken the time to evaluate her situation and kindly write up her story in the form of a poem using an analogy situation, which we feel beautifully draws the picture in a way that most people can understand. The first part of the poem begins the journey through this book, and there is a second part that helps to conclude our family perspective focus. Don't jump and read it just yet. Even though we know you will want to when you read part one, allow the poem to fill your mind with thoughts and questions, and allow the book to take you through some of our shared ideas, information and experiences.

'Welcome to Holland'

I am often asked to describe the experience of raising a child with a disability – to try to help people who have not shared that unique experience to understand it, to imagine how it would feel. It's like this...

When you're going to have a baby, it's like planning a fabulous vacation trip – to Italy. You buy a bunch of guide books and make your wonderful plans. The Coliseum. The Michelangelo David. The gondolas in Venice. You may learn some handy phrases in Italian. It's all very exciting.

After months of eager anticipation, the day finally arrives. You pack your bags and off you go. Several hours later, the plane lands. The stewardess comes in and says, 'Welcome to Holland.'

'Holland?!' you say. 'What do you mean Holland?? I signed up for Italy! I'm supposed to be in Italy. All my life I've dreamed of going to Italy.'

But there's been a change in the flight plan. They've landed in Holland and there you must stay.

The important thing is that they haven't taken you to a horrible, disgusting, filthy place, full of pestilence, famine and disease. It's just a different place.

So you must go out and buy new guide books. And you must learn a whole new language. And you will meet a whole new group of people you would never have met.

It's just a different place. It's slower-paced than Italy, less flashy than Italy. But after you've been there for a while and you catch your breath, you look around… and you begin to notice that Holland has windmills… and Holland has tulips. Holland even has Rembrandts.

But everyone you know is busy coming and going from Italy… and they're all bragging about what a wonderful time they had there. And for the rest of your life, you will say 'Yes, that's where I was supposed to go. That's what I had planned.'

And the pain of that will never, ever, ever, ever go away… because the loss of that dream is a very very significant loss.

But… if you spend your life mourning the fact that you didn't get to Italy, you may never be free to enjoy the very special, the very lovely things… about Holland.

Emily Perl Kingsley, 1987

Reproduced with our acknowledgement, respect and gratitude – Julie Adams and Diana Leshone.

Chapter 1

Legislative frameworks for supporting children with disabilities

It is easy to be confused by legislation when working in any sector of social work, particularly when the legislation (law) is then interpreted into our policies and procedures. We are not going to give you every bit of legislation within this chapter; we aim to give you an *awareness* of a few of the recent changes, with a brief outline of some of the pertinent points. We are not giving legal advice and would always advise that YOU do not either, but instead talk to your legal department and always direct families to agencies that can offer them such advice. Also, please note we are referring to English legislation unless stated otherwise.

Remember that in some instances local authorities have a 'duty to act', meaning they must do something, and in other instances they have a 'power to act', which means that the law *enables* them to do a certain thing, but at their own discretion.

The Care Act 2014

The Care Act 2014 received Royal Assent on 14 May 2014. This means it is now law. The principle of the legislation is to promote 'well-being', including dignity, physical and mental health, protection from abuse and neglect, having control over day-to-day life and being able to participate in education and/or training. The main focus of the Act is on adults, see www.communitycare.co.uk/2007/01/05/direct-payments-personal-budgets-and-individual-budgets/. The Act promotes these principles both for the carer and for the person with care needs.

In relation to the transition to adult services, under the Act, an adult carer is:

an adult (including one who is a parent of the child) who provides or intends to provide care for the child (Department of Health 2014: clause 60 s(7)).

A young carer is defined as:

a person under 18 who provides or intends to provide care for an adult (DH 2014 (c23): clause 63 s(6)).

Consideration should be given by the local authority as to whether to refer the young carer for a young carer's assessment, an assessment of need under the Children Act 1989, or a young carer's assessment under Section 63 of the Care Act. Both adult and children's services need to be working together to ensure both the adult's and child's needs are being met (DH 2014b: para 6.68:89).

The assessment of the young carer should take into account factors such as:

> » is their caring role appropriate?
>
> » what tasks are they doing in this role and are they excessive?
>
> » what is the impact upon their health, emotional and physical development and well-being?
>
> » is their education and learning being affected?
>
> » what are the young carer's views about their caring role?

A carer has the right to have an assessment in their own right even if the person they are caring for refuses an assessment; however, a carer can also refuse to have an assessment. The local authority must consider any services being provided to the carer under Section 17 of the Children Act 1989 (DH 2014 (c23): clause 62(3):53).

Clause 12 of the Act states that the assessments must have regard to the needs of the 'whole family'. The whole family approach should in principle allow each individual family member to have their wishes and aspirations considered and, at the same time, the strengths of the family as a unit to be taken into account within the family assessment. This approach also allows the family to only have to 'tell their story' once. A local authority can combine transition assessments for carers and people with care needs with any other assessments that are being carried out if the person to whom the assessment relates agrees (DH 2014 (c23): clause 65(1) to (5):56). This allows for a holistic, joint approach to assessments, which is in everyone's interest. Transition assessments could also potentially become part of a child or young person's Education, Health and Care (EHC) Plan.

The Care Act must consider if the child, young carer or adult caring for a child is likely to have needs when they, or the child they are caring for, turns 18 years of age. The young person or their carer may request an assessment for the young person who is approaching their 18th birthday regardless of whether they are currently in receipt of services. This is known as a 'transition assessment' (DH 2014 (c23): clause 60(6):52). We discuss the transition to adulthood further at the end of this chapter.

The Care Act 2014 provides continuity so that where a young person is receiving children's services, those services are not stopped as soon as they turn 18, but instead are continued until adult services has a plan in place or 'relevant steps' have been taken. In the authors' experiences, this should be a welcome addition to the current transition, when young people have had services end upon their 18th birthday and the transition to adult care has not, for various reasons, perhaps run smoothly. The impact upon the young adult can be great.

Under the Carers (Recognition and Services) Act 1995, adults that are caring for a disabled child but that do not have parental responsibility are entitled to an assessment to provide, or to continue to provide, care for the disabled child. Consideration must be given to the carer's wishes to work, or to engage in recreation activities or training or education.

The Children Act 1989

It is likely that you are familiar with the Children Act 1989 and how the Act underpins most of the work you do with children and young people. The Children Act 1989 places a duty on local authorities to *'promote and safeguard the welfare of children in their area'* (Department for Education 2015:96). This is briefly covered in Chapter 6 in the context of assessments.

The definition of children in need includes children who are disabled within the meaning of the 1989 Act. Section 17(11) states: *'...a child is disabled if he is blind, deaf or dumb or suffers from mental disorder of any kind or is substantially and permanently handicapped by illness, injury or congenital deformity...'* (Department for Children, Schools and Families 2010a:7).

Section 17: explores children's needs under a 'children in need' basis. A child in need is defined under the Act as a child who is *'unlikely'* to achieve or *'maintain a reasonable level of health or development',* or *'whose health and development is likely to be significantly or further impaired without the provision of services'.* By virtue of being a *'child who is disabled'* that child is a 'child in need' (DCSF 2010:35).

Section 17 of the Children Act 1989 states that local authorities are responsible for determining which services should be provided to a child in need; however, this does not mean that the local authority necessarily has to provide the services itself.

From 1 April 2015, provisions relating to young carers and parent carers have been inserted into Part 3 of the Children Act (1989) by Sections 96 and 97 of the Children and Families Act 2014.

Section 47: Under Section 47 the local authority has a duty to make enquiries when there is reasonable cause to suspect that a child (or children) is suffering or are likely to suffer *'significant harm'.* The local authority must decide what action is required in order to safeguard and promote the child's welfare (DCSF 2009: 42). We discuss safeguarding children with disabilities further in Chapter 2.

Section 31: deals with care orders (Section 38 for interim care orders). When a child is subject to a care order the local authority takes on the role of 'corporate parent' and shares parental responsibility for the child's needs. The child will have a care plan that sets out the services to be provided; it is regularly reviewed.

Section 20: gives the *'duty to accommodate a child'* if there is no one with parental responsibility to look after them, they are lost or abandoned, or because the person caring for them has been prevented from providing suitable accommodation or care. A child accommodated under Section 20 is cared for under voluntary care (DCSF 2010a). We will discuss some of the duties under Section 20 in more detail when looking at Short Breaks Regulations, namely Breaks for Carers of Disabled Children Regulations 2011, which came into effect in April 2011.

Children and Families Act 2014

The Children and Families Act was given Royal Assent on 22 April 2014, although some aspects of the Act did not come into force until a little later. The Act covers both private and public children's proceedings. The Act has brought about a wide range of reforms for vulnerable children; however, our main focus is on the changes for those children with special educational needs and disabilities (SEND).

Part 3 of the Act contains provisions following the green paper *Support and aspiration: a new approach to special educational needs and disability*, published by the DfE in March 2011, and the follow-up *Progress and next steps*, published in May 2012.

Part 3 of the Children and Families Act 2014 is entitled 'Children and Young People in England with Special Educational Needs and Disabilities'. It places duties on local authorities and other services in relation to both disabled children and young people and those with special educational needs (SEN), although not all the sections of the Act apply to both groups. Here, we aim to give you an overview of the SEND process, but suggest you consult the guidance document *Special educational needs and disability code of practice: 0 to 25 years – Statutory guidance for organisations which work with and support children and young people who have special educational needs or disabilities* (January 2015) for further reading.

The SEND Code of Practice 2015 states that a child or young person has SEN if they have *'a learning difficulty or disability which calls for special educational provision to be made for him or her'* (p 15 xiii). 'Special educational provision', for a child aged two or over, is provision that is *'additional to or different from that made generally for other children or young people of the same age by mainstream schools, maintained nursery schools, mainstream post-16 institutions or by relevant early years providers'* (p 16 para xv).

Local offer

Under the SEND reforms each local authority must be able provide information about what local services (health, care and education) are available for all families with children with SEND. They must have a 'Local Offer'. The SEND Local Offer should make it easier for families to find out what information is available to their family, giving a clear description of what help, support and services are available for children and young people with SEND, including the preparation for adulthood (up to age 25) in their local area (DfE and DH 2015).

Local authorities must also provide a description of the educational and training provisions that children and young people with special educational needs and/or disabilities can expect to be provided. This includes provision from early years, schools and post-16 provision. Schools must develop and provide detailed information that shows their arrangements for identifying, assessing and making provision available for their children with SEN (DH 2014c).

Concerns about a child or young person's SEN are often first identified in their education setting, which may be, for example, when they are attending nursery or a childminder's (known as Early Years), within their school setting, or even within a further educational setting such as college. If a child has a learning disability their SEN can be met either within a mainstream setting with extra support being provided or in a specialist educational school. The SEND regulations aim to ensure that any additional support a child requires is provided within their setting. It is important that once it has been identified that a child requires additional support, the setting discuss this with the parents, or persons with parental responsibility, in order to put a plan in place to ensure that the child is provided with 'early help'.

Under the legislation 'a child' is a person under compulsory school age, and the definition of a 'young person' is a person over compulsory school age, which is after the last day of the summer term when the person becomes 16 years of age (section 83(2)), but still under the age of 25. If the young person is deemed to have 'capacity' under the Mental Capacity Act 2005, they are entitled to make decisions regarding their SEND on their own behalf rather than a parent taking that decision (DfE and DH 2015: para 2.12:32 and para 8.19:128).

Graduated approach

'Early help' is additional support and provision that is available before any formal assessment. This system of early help and support is known as a 'Graduated Approach'. The support provided at this point is provided under 'SEN support', which replaced what was previously known as School Action and School Action Plus.

The Graduated Approach involves the Special Educational Needs Co-ordinator (SENCO), in consultation with others, assessing what help and support the child requires (*assess*) in order to co-ordinate planned provision (a *plan*) to ensure that the child's needs and agreed outcomes continue to be met. The teacher at the setting will put the agreed provision in place (*do*) with assistance from the SENCO, and they can track the child's progress and review the planned provision and make changes as required (*review*). If the child is not progressing further support may be requested from other professionals, for example speech and language therapists (SALT), occupational therapists (OT) or physiotherapists. This is a 'four-part cycle': ASSESS, PLAN, DO, REVIEW (DfE and DH 2015: para 7.15–7.21).

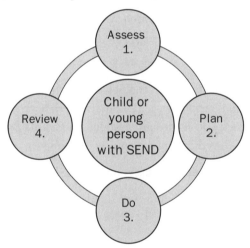

When a school is supporting a child with SEN, they can access monies from a 'notional budget' held by the school. The maximum mandatory cost threshold (at the time of writing) is £6,000. This money is to contribute towards the SEN support arrangements made by the school to support children with SEN and/or disabilities. Evidence of how this budget has been used would need to be provided when requesting an EHC Needs Assessment (Education Funding Agency 2014). There are many complexities and rules around funding matters, and different authorities may have different approaches, therefore we suggest you explore these issues depending on any specifics you wish to know about.

SENCO

What is a SENCO? All qualified teachers will at different times be involved with teaching children with SEN, but the SENCO is instrumental in developing early intervention strategies, carrying out assessments and giving advice about alternative strategies to support a child or young person's additional needs/requirements as they progress through their education. In a college setting, there will be a named person who has an oversight of the SEN provision in order to ensure that the young person's needs are co-ordinated. The Children and Families Act 2014 states '*the appropriate authority must designate a member of staff at the school, to be known as the "SEN co-ordinator", as having responsibility for co-ordinating the provision for pupils with special educational needs*' (DH 2014c:c6 s67:49).

The Special Educational Needs and Disability Regulations 2014 state that SENCOs have a legal duty for '*promoting the pupil's inclusion in the school community and access to the school's curriculum, facilities and extra-curricular activities*' (Statutory Instruments 2014: 1530 Part 3, p 24 c50 3(b) viii). They also highlight that a SENCO will:

- » Advise on the Graduated Approach
- » Liaise with the setting in order to inform/support how the setting's resources can be used to effectively meet the additional needs of the child
- » Liaise with educational psychologists, health professionals such as SALTs and OTs, Child and Adolescent Mental Health Services (CAMHS) and community nurses, social care professionals such as social workers, and other voluntary bodies that may be required for support
- » Ensure the educational setting is putting SEN policies in place effectively
- » Collaborate with curriculum co-ordinators at the setting to ensure that the learning requirements of all children with SEN are given equal emphasis and priority

Education, Health and Care Plan (EHCP)

A child with more complex needs might require an Education, Health and Care Plan (EHC Plan). The EHC Plans replace Statements of Special Educational Needs and Learning Disability Assessments (LDAs).

When requesting an EHC Needs Assessment, the setting will have to ensure that it has collated all its evidence from the four-part cycle (Graduated Approach of Assess, Plan, Do and Review). The setting has to be able to show how it has supported the child and what interventions have been utilised using the allocated supports provided for each child under the graduated approach prior to any assessment via the EHC route. An EHC Needs Assessment examines a child or young person's education, health and social care needs (DfE and DH 2015:86–87). Once it is felt that an application for assessment is required the local authority has to consider whether to carry out an EHC assessment within six weeks of receiving the request (relevant legislation: Section 36 of the Children and Families Act 2014, Regulations 3, 4 and 5 of the SEND Regulations 2014 and para 9.11 Code of Practice). If the local authority decides NOT to carry out an EHC assessment, the parent or young person can appeal using the First-tier (SEND) Tribunal procedure. Prior to this, however (and at other stages of the process where there is a disagreement), they must have considered mediation (para 9.57 and 9.126) and their right to, and the availability of, information, advice, support and disagreement resolution services.

If it is decided to progress with the EHC assessment, the local authority has a further ten weeks to undertake the assessment process (also known as a 'statutory assessment') to ascertain if the child requires an EHC Plan (Section 37(1)). The local authority must inform the young person or parent within 16 weeks of the original request for an EHC Needs Assessment if they are not progressing to an EHC Plan, and again there is a right to appeal the decision via the SEND Tribunal. The local authority has to decide whether the child or young person's needs can be met sufficiently via their Local Offer, SEN support/graduated approach. If a decision is made to progress to an EHC Plan, the local authority will liaise with the young person and/or family to discuss a suitable educational placement for the child or young person before naming the provision on the plan. The whole process must be completed within 20 weeks (DfE and DH 2015).

As stated in the name of the plan, the health and social care needs of the child must also be considered. Section 42(2) requires the responsible commissioning body to arrange the healthcare provision specified in the EHC Plan. Section 37(2) requires the local authority to identify any social care services for a child or young person (under 18 years of age) under the Chronically Sick and Disabled Persons Act 1970.

EHC Plans are reviewed at least annually (Section 44) to ensure that the provision identified in the plan continues to meet the child or young person's SEN and to check progress is being made to achieve outcomes. A young person's transition planning should start during Year 9 of school, when the child will be 13 or 14 years old, as a statutory requirement, and this extends until the child is 25 years of age. The focus of the plan is on the young person's preparation towards adulthood. Good practice would suggest that using the Transition Pathway would help any young person regardless of them having a Pathway Plan (under the looked-after children system) or an EHC Plan.

The plan can be ended (Section 45) when it is felt there is no longer a need or the local authority is no longer responsible for the child or young person (DfE and DH 2015).

Here is a *very* simple flow chart of the EHC process.

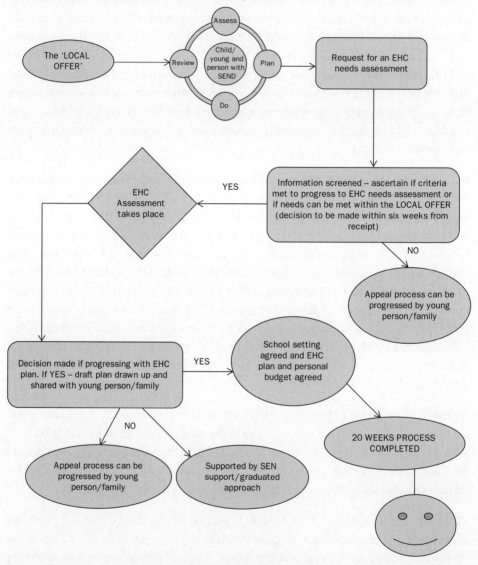

Note: There are 'infographs' available online that show you some of the step-by-step diagrams of the processes for the SEND reforms, which may be helpful for you or for you to direct families to: www.specialneedsjungle.com/new-send-system-f low-charts-together/.

Once it has been agreed that the local authority is progressing with an EHC Plan, the young person and family will be invited to apply for a 'Personal Budget' under Section 48 of the Act. The personal budget is the amount identified as available to secure the particular provisions set out in the EHC Plan, and can take the form of a direct payment, with the family being able to spend the monies as a cash amount, or a notional budget held by the local authority, or a combination of the two.

Personal budgets and direct payments are discussed further at the end of this chapter.

Chronically Sick and Disabled Persons Act (CSDPA) 1970

The CSDPA applies equally to both children and adults and, in addition, the National Service Framework (NSF) also relates to disabled children, specifically when looking at 'equipment and adaptations', highlighting that consideration should be given by local authorities to disabled children, young people and their families' housing and equipment (including wheelchair) needs to maximise their health and well-being. Furthermore, any equipment and assistive technology they require should be accessible in all settings (DH 2004).

Assessments that are undertaken for equipment and/or adaptations, ie for a Disabled Facilities Grant, are undertaken under the CSDPA and are usually completed by an occupational therapist.

When undertaking an assessment of a child with a disability, the local authority must also consider whether it is necessary to provide support under Section 2 of the Act. Where a local authority is satisfied that the identified services and assistance can be provided under Section 2, and it is necessary in order to meet a disabled child's needs, it must arrange to provide that support (DfE 2015:18).

Section 2 of the CSDPA is concerned with the provision of welfare services; however the Children Act 1989 is the statutory framework that underpins local authorities' responsibilities for children and their families. Disabled children and their families that are provided with services under the CSDPA are still assessed for that need under Part 3 of the Children Act 1989; disabled children are deemed to be 'children in need' under Section 17. Prior to making the final decision about providing and agreeing services, the local authority should consider if their criteria give consideration to the CSDPA.

The collaboration between the CSDPA and the Children Act is not easy.

The Mental Capacity Act 2005

The Mental Capacity Act (MCA) relates to England and Wales. It applies to adults and to young people aged 16 and over. Examples of those who may have difficulty making decisions are people with a learning difficulty, mental health problem, brain injury, dementia or who have had a stroke.

Section 1 of the MCA has five main principles that are specifically designed to protect those people who lack the capacity to make particular decisions in their life. In addition, the Act also helps promote a person's independence in that it assists them to be able to make some decisions, or to participate in decision-making regarding their life as far as they are able to do so. It is important to remember that anyone you are supporting is entitled to make decisions, regardless of whether you think it is a bad or unwise one. We should not take the view that because their decision is unwise they do not have the capacity to make that decision. As a social worker you should ensure that the person is allowed to make their decision by being given the correct information, and in doing so, they must have understanding about the decision they are making and its implications. A person should not be treated as being unable to make a decision unless all practicable steps have been taken to help them. If you are making a decision for a person, or have already made that decision for someone who lacks capacity, it must be done in the person's best interests. In the first instance, however, the MCA starts with the premise that a person who is making the decision '*must be assumed to have the capacity unless it is established that he/she lacks capacity*' (Department of Constitutional Affairs 2005 (c9):1).

When assessing a person's mental capacity there is a two-stage test for considering if a person has the capacity to make a decision (DCA 2007:44–45). This test asks:

Stage 1: Does the person have an impairment of, or a disturbance in the functioning of, their mind or brain? (Evidence must be provided);

Stage 2: Does the impairment or disturbance mean that the person is unable to make a specific decision when they need to? (Evidence must be provided).

It asks the questions, can the person:

    (a)   understand the information relevant to the decision?

    (b)   retain that information?

    (c)   use or weigh that information as part of the process of making the decision?

    (d)   communicate his/her decision (whether by talking or any other means)?

You may find that when you are working with a young person there is a conflict between what the young person wants to do in their life and what their parent feels is appropriate. This is when you may use the MCA to help assess whether the young person has the 'capacity' to make the decision about what they want to do. A young person may not be able to decide about the major decisions in their life, for example money matters or about important medical treatment, but they can perhaps make decisions about how they decorate their bedroom, or whom they wish to allow into their home etc. Being unable to make some decisions does not make a person unable to make all the decisions in their life. It is also important to note that capacity needs to be considered by asking one particular question at a time. Basically the whole concept would need to be broken down into specific questions about each aspect before a decision about capacity to consent can be considered.

Consider the MCA in this real context.

Scenario: Going on the train

Jeffery is 17 years old and has severe autism. He lives at home with his mother. Jeffery has an obsession with trains and visiting train stations and makes lots of schedules about which train stations he wants to visit and when. This affects Jeffery's family and he controls a lot of what the family can do and where they can go. If Jeffery does not get to go where he wants, he is sometimes aggressive and will hit out and hurt family members if they try and stop him. Carers work with Jeffery and take him out into the community and to different train stations to watch the trains and make train journeys. They also work with Jeffery to try and help him understand that although his schedules are important to him, they are at times unrealistic and his family cannot always take him to the stations he wants to go to – and that he must not hurt his family because of this. Jeffery is determined that when he is 18, he wants to go to the station and go on a train on his own. Jeffery's mother does not want him to do this. She is afraid he would not understand the risks in the community, and that he could get into difficult situations while on the train due to not understanding the social cues of other passengers or staff.

On the occasions when Jeffery has hurt his family the police have sometimes been called and Jeffery has been taken to the police station. The police, however, deemed that Jeffery did not have the 'capacity' to be charged for breach of the peace or assault. Because Jeffery was so challenging, a lot of support had to be

> *put in place to help manage his behaviours, but it was not possible to have staff in Jeffery's home all the time. The situation was very difficult to manage.*
>
> Think about the scenario – what are the issues you would consider with regard to Jeffery's capacity to make his own decisions? What decisions would you allow him to make? Do you think Jeffery should be able to travel on the train alone? If so, what measures would you put in place to help Jeffery achieve his wish to travel on the train alone? How might you stop Jeffery assaulting his family?
>
> Also consider that principle 5 of the MCA states that before a decision is made *'regard must be given to whether the purpose for which it is needed can be as effectively achieved in a way that is less restrictive of the person's rights and freedom of action'* (DCA 2005: (c9):1(6):2).

Advocacy

Advocacy is the process undertaken to help a person express their wishes, feelings and views, and to ensure their rights and best interests are taken into consideration and represented. The Advocate's role is to ensure that the 'child's voice' is heard and listened to, and to help a person be aware of the different options and choices available to them. Although you in your role as a social worker must advocate for the child, there are times when there are conflicts of interest in your professional role (for example, when working with other colleagues in health or adult social care who have different professional agendas), or you are in conflict with the parents' wishes and feelings about their child's best interests. It is important therefore to think about when a child or young person should have an independent advocate. Just before reading on, think about which decisions may require an advocate?

Independent advocates are often allocated to children and young people (with or without learning difficulties) when there is to be a Child Protection Case Conference, including at Conference Review, and when a child is a looked-after child. They have to be skilled in communicating with children with additional needs in order to be able to achieve their wishes and consider their feelings, and to support them at meetings or to advocate on their behalf should they choose not to attend or are unable to attend their meeting.

We recommend you read The Bournewood Judgment, a ruling made by the European Court of Human Rights in HL v UK (2004), amended by the Mental Health Act 2007, and *Deprivation of Liberty Safeguards (DoLS)*.

Short Breaks for Carers of Disabled Children Regulations 2011

The Short Breaks for Carers of Disabled Children Regulations came into effect in April 2011.

It is clearly documented (DCSF 2009) that the parents and siblings of disabled children are under a significant amount of stress due to having to manage the complex care needs of those children. These families also present more often in the lower levels of parental well-being and poverty groups due to many parents being unable to work, or having reduced working hours, due to the care needs of their disabled child. Furthermore, disabled children are three to four times more likely than non-disabled children to be abused or neglected, and to suffer bullying and mental health disorders. In order for families to be able to manage and continue to meet the care needs of the disabled child, and to keep families together, it is essential that they are given the opportunity to 'recharge their batteries' and that provision is put in place to safeguard children with disabilities and their families. It has been recognised therefore that there is a need for short breaks.

Aiming High for Disabled Children (DCSF 2008a) contributed to the increase in short breaks now available. Short breaks are intended to benefit children and young people with a disability, including those with sensory impairments and complex health needs, and their families, by offering them positive and enjoyable experiences away from their primary carer. These breaks should at the same time offer the parent and/or carer time away from their caring responsibility. A 'Short Break' can take different formats, including:

» Daytime care, which can be in the disabled child's home or elsewhere

» Educational or leisure activities for the disabled child out of their own home

» After-school clubs, holiday clubs etc during evenings, weekends and school holidays

» Overnight care in the home or elsewhere.

The short break can be anything from just a few hours to a number of days or a weekend, and can include overnight breaks. The 'setting' for this can be: 'Universal' ie, accessible to everyone within the community, for example a sports club or a youth club; 'Targeted', which would be aimed at children with disabilities or sensory needs and be provided by third party organisations such as after-school clubs, holiday clubs and/or buddying services; or 'Specialist', for those children and young people whose disability or sensory impairment requires a higher level of support.

Access to specialist services is via an Assessment of Need under the Children Act 1989. This assessment is often undertaken by social workers within Children with Disabilities teams. These specialist services may be provided within the home or outside of the home and can include overnight care dependent upon the assessed need.

The short break should also help the disabled child to:

» Build up their network of friendships

» Increase their independence skills

» Access leisure services

» Improve their levels of well-being and happiness, as well as those of their family

» Reduce the social isolation often associated with having disabilities

Under the Breaks for Carers of Disabled Children Regulations 2011 local authorities are legally bound to provide a range of short breaks for children aged 0–18 year old. Therefore, the Local Offer should set out the information and support services available for children and young people regarding the short breaks on offer within each local authority.

Some children with disabilities may receive a much higher level of short breaks than others, and therefore it is important that the level of review and safeguarding required is proportionate to the package that has been identified to meet the needs of the child and their family.

Overnight short breaks

Short breaks can be provided by local authorities under the Children Act 1989:

» Section 17(6) or;

» Section 20(4).

It is important that the local authority consider the legal basis for which a service is provided, and that as has already been discussed, any services are only provided following an assessment of the child's needs, considering all factors, including parenting capacity, family and environmental factors and the child's wishes and feelings (DfE 2011a).

Research undertaken by Radcliffe et al (2007) identifies a potential conflict of interest. It found that many disabled children on a respite break were distressed and homesick, but parents may not recognise such distress or its extent because of their own and the other family members' need for a break from their caring role. The research found those children suffering homesickness displayed anxiety, unhappiness and physical symptoms, including behavioural difficulties, being unsettled and frequently screaming leading up to a stay in respite and in the days following their return home. Those of you who are familiar with working with children with disabilities, however, will know that for some children with learning disabilities such as autism, the anxiety building up to respite, transitions to and from settings and/or the change in routine can bring on many of the behaviours described by Radcliffe. The DfE (2011a) stipulates that it is challenging for those families caring for children with complex health needs; challenging behaviour and profound disabilities, and their impact upon family life, must be an integral part of your assessment when considering short breaks. The local authority (you as a social worker) must also consider the impact of a child's disability upon their siblings, and the benefits to the non-disabled siblings of the respite (DfE 2011a). There are numerous investigations into the significant benefits of respite to parents and siblings (Byrne and Cunningham 1985; Robinson and Stalker 1990; Bose 1991; Hubert 1991; Chadwick et al 2002; MacDonald and Callery 2004; MacDonald et al 2007, cited in Radcliffe et al 2007:92).

A child's attachment does affect their experiences in care, and issues such as the regular turnover of staff can heighten a child's sense that they are not loved or wanted (Maclean and Harrison 2008:86). It is acknowledged that parents feel guilty for sending their child to respite, particularly if they suffer distress, but this has to be balanced with the difficulties and strains that go alongside bringing up a child with a disability. Langer et al (2010) stated that quality overnight respite care was pivotal to parents' ongoing ability to provide care to their disabled child. Finally, it is important that you think carefully about those young people who use short breaks and who are progressing towards adulthood, and the services that the young person may or may not be entitled to as an adult. For example, if a young person in children's services is receiving a high number of overnight short breaks and they are not likely to continue to receive a similar level of respite care in adult services, it would be sensible to start to reduce the amount of overnights leading up to the transition to Adult Social Care. Likewise, if a young person has been assessed in their seventeenth year by Adult Social Care to be moving forward, for example into a supported living environment, and they are only having overnights every few months, moving to a full-time supported living environment could prove difficult for the young person who is suddenly living away from home when they have not been used to spending time away from their parents/carers. Welch et al (2010:132) state that the transition period is often *'felt to be catastrophic by families as an array of family supports, including short breaks, are drastically reduced as their child officially becomes an adult'.*

Within a climate of financial restraint and government-enforced cuts, there are far more challenges that you as social workers must consider when a child has been assessed as having an unmet social care need for social inclusion. It can be difficult when you are considering which provision is able to meet that need, particularly when the family want overnight care and you as the assessing social worker may feel that it is not an 'assessed need'. Often the social worker may feel that the unmet need can actually be met via Universal services or a few hours' worth of direct payments, but the family feel that it can only be met via an overnight break. There is often disagreement between a 'want' and a 'need', and in the authors' experience, this may even result in parents making complaints when the outcome of the assessment is different to what they want or feel they are entitled to. You must not let this influence your assessment. Your recommendation must be drawn from your evidence – not because you may feel sorry for their situation or fear a complaint. Welch et al (2010:132) highlight that those families who have used short breaks are less likely to welcome and adopt direct payments or personalisation that could be used to effect such rebalancing.

It is essential therefore that once a young person is receiving a short break, you, as a social worker, are monitoring all of these issues, ie the type of respite care received, its effects, any changes in behaviour leading up to and after respite, the young person's transition towards adult social care and the needs of the parent(s), carers and any siblings. It is essential that all these issues are discussed openly in the child is review, concerns recorded and flexible, creative options for short breaks explored (Langer et al 2010).

When it has been assessed that the child should receive overnight short breaks, it must then be decided under which section of the Children Act 1989 the child should be accommodated (Section 17(6) or Section 20(4)). The number of nights and the frequency of the breaks are factors that will contribute to this decision. You must also consider whether the child is having an overnight short break in more than one setting, ie within a school or hospice, and how much contact they will have with their family during the break. The complexities of the situation will determine if the child is considered a looked-after child and if their care package is reviewed by an Independent Reviewing Officer (IRO) or a social worker.

There are circumstances where Section 20(4) has been modified to include Regulation 48; this covers children whose short breaks total fewer than 75 nights per year with no single placement lasting more than 17 nights (DCSF 2010a). Examples in brief:

Section 17(6): Eleanor has one overnight stay (less than a 24-hour period) per month at a local short breaks respite care unit. There are no concerns about the level of care Eleanor receives from her parents, and the care package was put in place to allow

Eleanor to experience greater social inclusion and to build her friendships, as well as to allow Eleanor's sibling Sophie to have time with her parents. The parents transport Eleanor to her short break.

This care package would most likely be reviewed by a social worker. There would be a child in need care plan.

Section 20(4): John is 15 years old and has autism, cerebral palsy and challenging behaviour. He has a younger sibling with additional needs, and two other siblings under five years of age, but they do not have any learning disabilities. It is very challenging for his parents to balance John's needs with the competing demands of his siblings and running the home, particularly as John's father works long shifts and is away from home two nights per week. John also has carers in the home to help with his personal care, which are provided by a direct payment. John has up to 12 overnights per year at the local hospice, and several overnights per month with a short breaks foster carer at her home; occasionally he also has emergency care when his parents are unable to manage his behaviour.

This care package would most likely be reviewed by an IRO and must have a looked-after child care plan.

Section 20(4), Regulation 48: Wendy lives at home with her mother and father. Wendy has Down's syndrome and is demanding of her parents' attention, which takes their time away from their two other children. Wendy can at times display challenging behaviour and sometimes gets up in the night, which means her mother also has to get up to ensure her safety. Wendy is 16 years old and enjoys attending a youth club, and she is working towards her independence skills for when she is 18 years old. It has been assessed that Wendy would benefit from regular prearranged short breaks one night a month and longer weekend breaks, which are prebooked and total fewer than 75 nights per year, at a local short breaks provider where she can be with her peer group.

This care package would likely be reviewed by an IRO and would have a short breaks care plan.

Statutory visits to children having overnight short breaks

As a social worker, there is an expectation that you will undertake statutory visits to children and young people whilst they are on their overnight short breaks. Each local authority may have 'good practice' policy and procedure guidance which has expectations that the visits are made more often than stipulated in the guidance. You should always read the policy and procedures of the organisation you work for.

There are different arrangements and conditions for children having short breaks and those children who are accommodated under Section 20(4). We recommend that you become familiar with the DCSF (2010a) 'Short Breaks Statutory Guidance' Chapter 2 and (DCSF 2010b) 'The Children Act 1989 Guidance and Regulations Volume 2: Care Planning, Placement and Case Review'.

Personal budgets and direct payments

Direct payments

Direct payments were first introduced in 1997 under the Community Care (Direct Payments) Act 1996. In 2001 the Carers and Disabled Children Act 2000 was introduced to include parents of disabled children and carers; this added a new Section 17A into the Children Act 1989. In 2009, provision was extended to persons appointed to receive direct payments on behalf of individuals who lack mental capacity and to persons subject to mental health legislation – Community Care, Services for Carers and Children's Services (Direct Payments) (England) Regulations 2009 (SI 2009/1887). The Care Act 2014 introduced the Care and Support (Direct Payments) Regulations 2014, which put personal budgets firmly into law for people with eligible assessed needs and carers, including the right to direct payment.

A direct payment is a different method families can choose as an alternative to services provided by Social Care, in other words they are 'in lieu' of services that would be provided under Section 17 of the Children Act 1989. Prior to any direct payment or personal budget being paid an assessment of need must be completed. It is worth noting here that assessments are not undertaken to assess for direct payments, but to assess a child or young person's unmet needs. As a result of the assessment and an identified unmet need, the local authority may offer a direct payment.

Parents (or a person with parental responsibility) or young people 16 years or over and up to 18 years of age can choose to employ a personal assistant (PA) and are responsible for all obligations as an 'employer'. This involves the parent being responsible for aspects associated with employment law, such as having a job description for the PA and managing their tax, national insurance and holiday pay. Direct payments must be paid into a separate bank account and the person managing the payments on behalf of the child is responsible for ensuring that they can provide evidence of how the monies have been used. Payroll agencies can support with Her Majesty's Revenue and Customs (HMRC) and some people may have a supported or 'managed account' provider, which will provide a person who works on the parents' behalf to manage the administrative responsibilities of the direct payment account. Some of these providers will also help with advertising for the PA etc. The direct payment account holder will still hold the employer responsibilities and have to ensure that they provide time sheets etc to the account manager. The direct payment should be sufficient to meet the service user's eligible needs and must be spent on services that meet those needs. The direct payment should form part of the child in need plan and will be reviewed on a regular basis alongside other identified needs.

When a parent has made the decision to use direct payments either to employ a PA or purchase services from a registered provider, the local authority retain their responsibilities under the Children Act 1989 to assess and review the needs of the disabled child and their family (DH 2009:para 163).

There are many rules associated with direct payments, such as not being allowed to employ a family member living in the family home or an agency carer in which the family has a vested interest. We suggest you read the *DH Guidance on Direct Payments for Community Care, Services for Carers and Children's Services: England 2009* and updated guidance since the Care Act 2014 (principally for adults), Care and Support (Direct Payments) Regulations 2014.

Personal budgets

A personal budget may also be known as an 'individual budget' and again is only provided following an assessment of need, as a means to meet all or part of the assessed unmet need. The assessed person may choose to allow the local authority to commission services on their behalf, or have a cash amount as a direct payment to choose how their care needs are met, or a third-party arrangement where direct payments are paid and managed by a third party on behalf of the individual young person or their parent. In some instances, they may decide to have a combination of the above (DfE and DH 2015:3.38:48). Personal budgets have a wider scope within their use than direct payments.

As with direct payments, the service user will, where possible, be involved in contributing to their support plan with their social worker and their family, and the implementation of the plan (known as brokerage). The support plan will be reviewed in a timely fashion.

Under Care Act 2014 guidance, where it is identified to be in a person's best interest to combine a personal budget and direct payments because they are receiving support from partner organisations (ie, health budget and social care), and the person agrees, the plans can be combined and attempts made to co-ordinate payments to avoid multiple payments and accounts having to be managed. Consideration might be given to a 'lead organisation' overseeing the budget and monitoring the direct payments to ensure both health and care needs are being met, and that both agencies are continuing to meet their statutory responsibilities (DH 2014b:para 12.60:216). The authors believe that for some managers, who are protective and possibly bordering on possessive about their budgets, actually giving control of them over to another discipline or person would be very difficult. Therefore, this would need a more pragmatic approach, with new policies and procedures being introduced whereby health, adult and children's social care have a pooled budget, rather than the rigid processes that are currently in place and that add delays to assessed outcomes being agreed and implemented.

Equality Act 2010

The Equality Act covers many different aspects and we suggest you look at the Act more closely for any specific issues you want to find out about. Much of the Act focuses around adults; however, we felt it wise to draw your attention to issues surrounding the police, education and employment.

If a young person finds themselves being questioned by the police, the police must consider their disability. A person with a learning disability should have an appropriate adult with them to ensure their needs are being met and they are given a break if necessary. A person with speech difficulties, or deafness or a hearing impairment should be provided with an interpreter. The police can, however, for both of the above undertake the interviews if a delay would mean harm to people, places or property (www.gov.uk/guidance/equality-act-2010-guidance).

Under the Equality Act 2010, it is unlawful for an education establishment to treat disabled students unfavourably. This could be indirectly, for example, not providing an application form in large print for a person with a visual impairment, or directly, for example a school not allowing a student to attend because of their disability. The setting has to ensure they are not discriminating against a student due to their disability, for example they should not prevent a disabled child going on a school trip because of the additional time and effort it would take for them to get on and off the transport. The education setting has to be seen to make reasonable adjustment to meet the needs of the disabled student, such as making physical changes to the environment or providing specialist equipment to support the disabled person. Higher education settings should have a person available to support their disabled students. As stated in the SEND sections, all settings must try to assess and meet the needs of children with disabilities.

Finally, it is against the law for employers to discriminate against a person because of their disability. A person's disability has to be taken into consideration, for example with application forms, interviews and any tests that are part of the selection pro-cess. The employer must also consider terms of employment for the disabled person, and the rights extend to promotion and issues such as disciplinary procedures and grievances, dismissal or redundancy etc. Once again the employer needs to consider reasonable adjustments to ensure that the disabled person is not disadvantaged com-pared with non-disabled colleagues.

Transition to adulthood

All children have to manage the different transitions throughout their lives, whether it be the transition to nursery and then first school, or their first time away from home, perhaps going to university. Children with disabilities may have more chal-lenges along the way, however, particularly if they find the smallest of changes a traumatic experience. One of the biggest challenges is the move into adult services. This can be difficult for both the person experiencing the transition and for their parents and carers, who have often been worrying about this change since their child has been a young teenager. Many parents/carers worry about who will look after their child if they are not able to do so or when they are no longer around. When you are working with a young adult who is approaching this transition, there-fore, you need to remember that close family members will probably be in turmoil at different times.

When a young person reaches their 18th birthday there are challenges such as:

» the change to different health professionals. A child who has grown up and become familiar with their paediatric consultant, for example, who has a really good understanding and professional relationship with the child and family, will have to be transferred to adult services and a new consultant;

» those children with complex needs who are supported by continuing care will be reassessed under the adult criteria for planning their healthcare needs as they reach adulthood;

» a change of social worker, as children's teams usually end their involvement when the young person reaches their 18th birthday;

» this often being a time when families feel that they can no longer manage their disabled child at home. This is a natural time for young adults to 'fly the nest' and parents can accept their disabled child moving on when they are 18, or they may have struggled to cope for many years and this is the natural transition time for them.

With all these things going on, you can understand why this is a stressful time. On a positive note, many young people with disabilities do stay in their educational setting (as part of their EHC Plan) until they are 19 years old (or longer for some settings), before making their transition to higher education or adult settings. This means that they will often have the familiarity and routine of school, which will give them some consistency during this period of change.

So what might this transition look like?

As we said earlier, the SEND reforms have implemented a new approach that seeks to join up support across education, health and care, from birth to 25.

Before we go on to discuss what this might look like in more detail, we would like to remind you that each child's journey will be different, depending upon the extent of their complex health needs or disability. Not all young people will be able to live independently or enter the field of employment, with some requiring 24-hour care or similar. Nevertheless, each young person should have transition planning and be supported in meeting their aspirations, be valued, and the same processes should be followed as with any other young person with additional needs: each child's hopes and ambitions must be celebrated and strived for in the same way. The plan should consider the services that the young person will be eligible for and professionals should work together to ensure that a holistic plan is achievable.

Let's look at what Harry's transition may look like.

Scenario: Harry's journey

Harry has Down's syndrome and attends a special educational needs school. He is now reaching the crucial time for him to start making plans for his future. You might think that starting this at 14 is young, but it is important that Harry is given time to think about his aspirations and what he wants to do as he makes his journey into adulthood. The transition planning allows Harry to consider factors such as his employment, independent living, inclusion within his local community and any health needs. This process is also important as it gives time to those key people in Harry's life who are going to be helping support him in achieving a meaningful life. Everyone needs to have a shared understanding of Harry's wishes and how to help him achieve his aspirations. Because this planning is done over years it gives Harry time to think about what he is interested in and good at, what he wants to aspire to and how to help achieve his goal.

Let's look at Harry's time line:

While Harry is aged around 11 years old, in Year 6 at school, the school's staff would hold an informal discussion with Harry and his family (or carers) about his future transition, explaining what this means for Harry and offering some information and advice if Harry or his family need this.

Harry reaches his 14th birthday:

» During this year Harry will have a Year 9 Annual Review meeting at school, which will start to look at and explore Harry's hopes and plans for his future. Harry's EHC Plan would also be reviewed at this meeting (not all children will have an EHC Plan and the transition pathway could be used to help the child plan for their future).

» Harry would be supported to make his Person-Centred Plan so that he can use this to have something tangible that sets out, in a child-centred way, his future plans.

Harry reaches his 15th birthday:

» Harry is now in Year 10, when his Year 10 Annual Review will take place, again looking at his future plans. Once again his EHC Plan (or the Transitions Pathway if no EHC Plan) is reviewed. This review would focus upon what Harry might want to do from the age of 16, for example looking at supporting Harry to have some brief period of work experience while still at school and developing independence skills to help him use buses to get there or manage his money.

Harry reaches his 16th birthday:

» Harry has progressed to Year 11 and his Year 11 Annual Review will be more involved, exploring what options are available for Harry, such as moving to a college, staying in a sixth form or going on to start other forms of training or work – so long as that work has a learning element attached to it*. This would be a good time to look at what benefits Harry may be entitled to in his own right. It may be appropriate to look at applying for an 'appointee' with the Department of Work and Pensions to help support Harry with benefits. On some occasions the parent/carer's wishes may be different to what Harry may want, and although Harry may be able to make some decisions it may be necessary to have an advocate to support him to ensure that his voice is heard.

» Once again Harry's EHC Plan (or Transition Pathway Plan) will be reviewed at this meeting.

* Children can leave school on the last Friday in June if they will be 16 by the end of the summer holidays. They must then do one of the following until they're 18: stay in full-time education, eg at a college; start an apprenticeship or traineeship; or work or volunteer (for 20 hours or more per week) while in part-time education or training (www.gov.uk/know-when-you-can-leave-school).

Harry reaches his 17th birthday:

> » By now Harry should have a good idea of his plan and things should be start-ing to develop. Once again, if Harry has decided to stay at school, he would have his Year 12 Annual Review, including an EHC Plan update, or if Harry has decided to go to college or sixth form his EHC plan would be reviewed.

> » Harry is entitled to have a transitions assessment to ensure his needs will continue to be met when he becomes an adult. A transitions assessment would be completed by Adult Social Care, and look at assessing Harry's needs, but also his carers', to ensure that their own needs are met and thus they can continue to support Harry.

> » At this time it would be appropriate to look at what type of supported employment, job coaching, apprenticeship or internship may be avail-able. It would be important to ensure that Harry is supported to look at any changes to benefit entitlements upon his 18th birthday, as these may change depending on the choices Harry makes.

Harry reaches his 18th birthday and is now classed as an adult:

> » Harry will be experiencing more changes in his life. For example, all of Harry's health needs would now be met by adult health services and he would no longer see the paediatrician who he saw as a child. If Harry has a social worker, when he turns 18 he would transfer to a new social worker from Adult Social Care. Harry's planning will really be taking shape: he may decide to leave education or go to, or remain at college, university or go into employment (the difference now is that Harry does not legally have to be in any education or training). If Harry has stayed on at school he will have a Year 13 Annual Review and his EHC Plan (or Transition Pathway Plan) would be reviewed; it would also be reviewed if he has decided to go to col-lege. The difference now, however, is that if Harry was to access a university his EHC Plan would end.

Harry while he is 19–25 years of age:

If still in school Harry would now be in Year 14, and would have his Year 14 Annual Review. Should Harry decide he no longer wants to continue with his education the

EHC plan would end. While in education (not university), up to 25 years of age his EHC plan would continue to be reviewed. During this period Harry may, if he has not already done so, decide to live independently (albeit this may be supported living), and he may look at what employment is available to him, perhaps having already started something like a supported internship or some work experience while deciding what he wants to do longer term.

www.gov.uk/government/publications/support-and-aspiration-a-new-approach-to-special-educational-needs-and-disability-progress-and-next-steps

Supported internships and apprenticeships

It is very important that young people with additional needs are treated fairly and given the same opportunities to progress and have meaningful occupations. Having a 'good job' is not only good because it allows them to have paid employment at the same rate as their work colleagues, but it also gives the likes of Harry the opportunity to have independence, build their self-esteem, give them an earned wage, learn new skills and offer job satisfaction. In order for young people who have special educational needs or disabilities to have these opportunities and be given a fair chance at maintaining the job once in post, Supported Internships and Apprenticeships have been introduced.

Supported internship

From August 2013, 'all young people in full- or part-time education aged 16 to 19 (16 to 24 where the student has a Learning Difficulty Assessment or Education, Health and Care (EHC) plan) have been expected to follow a study programme – a coherent, personalised learning programme that offers breadth, depth and progression' (DfE 2014:6).

A supported internship is a study programme specifically aimed at young people with additional needs who want to move into employment but need extra support to allow them to do this. It is recognised that many young people with complex health needs or severe learning disabilities may never be able to do this, but it is essential that those young people with SEN who *are* able to are given the opportunities and support to be able to achieve their aspirations in employment. A supported internship is a structured study programme designed to allow young people with SEN and/or disabilities to achieve 'sustainable paid employment'. The internship will allow them to learn skills through work-based placements that where possible then lead to employment. The placements would usually be for up to a year, and would include the intern undertaking an unpaid work placement for at least six months; at the end of the placement it is hoped the intern would progress to paid employment, ideally with the same employer, or they would be supported to look for alternative employment. The study alongside this may include maths and English, which would increase their chances of maintaining sustainable employment in the future.

Supported internships are structured, and different to an apprenticeship or traineeship as the interns require a higher level of support while on the programmes and the programmes are longer. While an apprentice has to pass assessments and qualifications in order to complete their apprenticeship, with supported internships there are no entry or completion requirements and each intern has a tailored programme that will meet their individual needs as they progress through the programme, ie it is 'supported' (DfE 2014).

Apprenticeships

An apprenticeship is an opportunity for a young person (or adult) to undertake practical training in a job while simultaneously studying. An apprenticeship will allow the apprentice to work alongside experienced staff and at the same time learn new skills that are specific to the job. They can earn a wage and have paid holidays while gaining a qualification. Often the apprentice is released to attend a course of study, which might be one day a week at a local college for example. The apprenticeship may last anything from one to four years, depending on the subject area. In order to apply for an apprenticeship, the young person must be 16 or over and not be in full-time education.

Prior to attending an apprenticeship, a young person may want to look at attending a 'traineeship', which is a course designed to give them work experience and get them 'ready for work'; this can last for up to six months. There are eligibility criteria for both traineeships and apprenticeships.

(See www.gov.uk/apprenticeships-guide or www.gov.uk/find-traineeship.)

There are further considerations for those disabled children and young people in care who are making the transition to adulthood, and again, planning must start early. Please read DfE 2014a for further guidance: page 123 gives references and resources for support for looked-after children who are making the transition to adulthood.

Benefits advice

As a social worker it is not your role to give families benefits advice (or any legal advice) and it is advisable that you direct service users to the relevant Citizens Advice Bureau, Benefits Agency Office or online resources.

The most common benefit that families with children with disabilities will receive is the **Disability Living Allowance** (DLA). This is a tax-free benefit for children under 16 years of age who have difficulties walking or require more looking after than a child of the same age who does not have a disability. There are certain eligibility criteria. The mobility component consists of lower and higher rates depending on the child's ability, the level of support they require to walk and discomfort experienced.

There is also a care component attached to the benefit and this also has different rates (low, middle and high), depending on the frequency of help required, level of supervision and if this includes night care, and also if the person has a terminal illness.

A parent or a person who cares for the child in the same way as if they were the child's parent can claim for DLA for the child they look after. There are special rules for children with a terminal illness. The benefit will be subject to assessment and reassessment.

Personal Independence Payments (PIP) started to replace the DLAs from 8 April 2013, and are tax-free payments for people with disabilities or long-term health conditions aged 16–64. There are different rates of payment dependent upon the severity of the condition, and the benefit is subject to assessment, with regular reassessment.

Carer's Allowance: A person may be eligible to claim a carer's allowance if they are 16 years of age or over and spend 35 hours or more per week caring for someone. There are other eligibility criteria, and some other benefits may exempt the person receiving them from being able to claim a Carer's Allowance. The person they are caring for must also be in receipt of certain benefits before the carer is eligible to claim a Carer's Allowance.

Employment and Support Allowance (ESA): A person may get ESA if their illness or disability affects their ability to work. A person who is employed, unemployed or a student who claims DLA or PIP may apply for ESA. If a person undergoes a Work Capability Assessment and is found eligible for work, in most cases they would not be eligible to put in a repeat claim for ESA, unless their condition has deteriorated or they have developed a new condition. A person may be able to claim ESA if they are doing 'supported permitted work', and there is no limit to the number of hours a person can work when doing such work, unlike those who are not supported.

We hope you found this chapter a useful guide to some of the important legislation and guidance that will help guide you in your practice while working with children with disabilities and their families. We hope by reading our 'Taking it further' section overleaf you will be ready for the challenges ahead. Remember, you are not a legal advisor and you should not give legal advice to families, but you can direct them to other agencies where they can get help. Always seek advice from your own legal team where necessary – but you usually need consent from your manager as it can be costly!

Taking it further

To find out more about the Mental Health Capacity Act visit The Office of the Public Guardian webpages at www.publicguardian.gov.uk

Further reading on the Children and Families Act 2014 on the Department for Education's website www.gov.uk/dfe or on the Parliament website

http://services.parliament.uk/bills/2013–14/childrenandfamilies.html and www.legislation.gov.uk/ukpga/2014/6/contents/enacted.

Hatton, C et al (2011) *The impact of short breaks on families with a disabled child over time: The second report from the quantitative study.* London: DfE.

Department for Children, Schools and Families (2010) *Short Breaks Statutory Guidance on how to safeguard and promote the welfare of disabled children using short breaks: England.* London: DCSF.

Department of Constitutional Affairs (2007) *Mental Capacity Act 2005 Code of Practice.* Birmingham: Office of the Public Guardian Chapter 4. Available online www.gov.uk/government/uploads/system/uploads/attachment_data/file/224660/Mental_Capacity_Act_code_of_practice.pdf.

The Sutton Trust-EEF Teaching and Learning Toolkit is an accessible summary of educational research, which provides guidance for teachers and schools on how to use their resources to improve the attainment of disadvantaged pupils:

Higgins, S, Katsipataki, M, Kokotsaki, D, Coleman, R, Major, L E and Coe, R (2014) *The Sutton Trust-Education Endowment Foundation Teaching and Learning Toolkit.* London: Education Endowment Foundation. Available online www.suttontrust.com/about-us/education-endowment-foundation/teaching-learning-toolkit/ (accessed 1 December 2015).

More additional reading:

H M Government Support and aspiration: A new approach to special educational needs and disability – consultation www.gov.uk/government/publications/support-and-aspiration-a-new-approach-to-special-educational-needs-and-disability-consultation (accessed 1 December 2015).

Social Care Institute for Excellence Adult carer transition in practice under the Care Act 2014 (2015) www.scie.org.uk/care-act-2014/transition-from-childhood-to-adulthood/adult-carer-transition-in-practice/index.asp (accessed 5 December 2015).

This chapter gives an overview, and explains the concepts, of safeguarding children with a disability but it is not an A-Z of safeguarding procedures. Each local authority and team has their own policies, procedures and training around safeguarding children. We are going to get you to think about some of the issues that relate to safeguarding children with disabilities and their additional vulnerabilities. Flowcharts of a generic Child Protection Section 47 process and the Child in Need Section 17 process showing the routes that a case may travel are included, as is a very brief explanation of what a Child Protection Case Conference and a Core Group is all about. We will look at Child in Need Meetings and how there are often additional complexities due to the child's disability. The role of the Independent Reviewing Officer is also explained.

We have given you definitions of when a child is deemed to be a 'child in need' under Section 17 of the Children Act 1989, or if a child is deemed to be 'at risk of significant harm' under Section 47 of the Children Act 1989 within Chapter 1. Remember, however, that a child with a disability is already deemed to be a child in need under Section 17 of the Children Act by virtue of having a disability. Within this book we have also used the term 'disabled child', which is taken from the relevant research or legislation.

Children with disabilities – the myths explored

It is important to remember that our personal beliefs (attitudes and assumptions) affect child protection, particularly those about disabled children, and that minimising the impact of abuse can lead to the failure to report abuse or neglect (DCSF 2009). It is frightening that despite media attention about abuse, society in general still seems to be in denial about the fact that disabled children are more likely to be abused than non-disabled children... Less attention is paid to their human rights... They are still commonly seen largely in terms of their 'impairment' (Stuart and Baines 2004: p 21).

Merchant (1991:pp 22–24) identified five myths about the sexual abuse of children with disabilities:

> » They are not vulnerable to sexual abuse.

> » You can't stop sexual abuse to disabled children happening.

> » If a disabled child has been abused, it is better to 'leave well alone' once they are safe.

> » It is OK to sexually abuse disabled children as it is not as harmful as abusing a non-disabled child.

> » Children with disabilities are more likely to make false allegations about abuse.

Such attitudes and myths can also lead to institutional abuse. Mencap discuss institutional discrimination and how they believe inadequate responses from health services leads to discrimination against people with learning disabilities. The report states people with learning disabilities are not equally valued within the health service, and staff who work within it often do not understand the needs of people with learning disabilities, which leads to their needs not being met (Mencap 2007: 6). Subsequently the investigation into the 2013 death of Connor Sparrowhawk, while he was a patient at a learning disability short-term assessment and treatment unit (part of Southern Health in Oxfordshire), concluded that the key issue in Connor's care was poor practice by clinical staff and that his death was preventable (Bartlett et al 2015).

Although we are not suggesting that malpractice is widespread within the health profession, it is essential that as a social worker you appropriately challenge professionals from *any* discipline if you are concerned about their attitudes and practices to avoid institutional abuse – be it intentional or unintentional.

The authors have experienced difficult discussions with police colleagues when undertaking Section 47 strategy meetings regarding concerns about disabled children being abused, and when comments have been made about whether a disabled child is a 'credible witness'. It is very frustrating when the police state that the case would not be pursued by the Crown Prosecution Service (CPS), as this makes you feel that they are of the opinion that the child with the disability is not worth the time and effort of an investigation. It is recognised however that there are complicating factors to be considered for children with disabilities. These could include:

> » Them being targeted by the perpetrator and frightened into secrecy

> » a delay in disclosure

> » the child being unaware that abuse has taken place

> » the child being viewed as fabricating the allegation

> » the child's account not being viable in the face of cross-examination from defence lawyers.

It is important to understand that the social worker's role is very different to that of the police. Police have to consider the issue of the prosecution finding evidence 'beyond all reasonable doubt' to secure a conviction against the perpetrator. When the police do not pursue a case it may not be because they do not believe that abuse has taken place, but due to the uncorroborated evidence of a child who is unable to give clear accounts of their abuse. If the defence can raise doubt in the jury's mind the defendant is entitled to be acquitted; judges are required to direct juries in criminal trials to return a verdict of not guilty if they are not 100% sure about the guilt of the defendant. In cases involving disabled children and young people as witnesses, the prosecution is bound by the same standard of proof as in any criminal trial (NSPCC 2003:69–70). If the child is put through the ordeal of giving evidence and it is unlikely to secure a conviction the police are less likely to go ahead. It is important to remember, however, that if the police are unable to secure a conviction or they do not believe a crime has been committed, social care can still take action, with the support of all agencies, against the perpetrator by instigating child protection policies and procedures (including legislation) to keep the child safe.

Safeguarding and child protection concerns for any child MUST be treated with the same professionalism and concern regardless of the child having a disability. If you come across a child being strapped to a chair for long periods of time and the parent says, 'It's for their safety so they don't fall or get into the cupboard to the bleach as they don't recognise danger', ask yourself 'Would I accept this answer for a non-disabled child?' 'NO.' The child is having their liberty restricted by being tied into their chair and you should consider the wider perspective, ask additional questions and not just accept that it must be alright as the child has a disability. You must see the child first and their disability must not deter you from considering child protection concerns. Also, where possible, communicate directly with the child or young person, using the most appropriate method of communication (see Chapter 4 for strategies to support you to do this).

We will explore an example later about a child who is locked into their bedroom and safeguarding considerations around this difficult issue. Many people will instantly recognise it as unacceptable, but there are occasions when it has been agreed as a last resort, with appropriate risk assessments.

Stalker et al (2010:4) in their research 'Child protection and the needs and rights of disabled children and young people: a scoping study' discuss the risk of practitioners applying higher thresholds to disabled children. They suggest that this is a result of over-identifying with the child's parents or carers and being reluctant to accept that abuse is taking place or seeing it as being attributable to the difficulties of caring for a disabled child. They state that:

» in Scotland, Wales, Northern Ireland and England the approach to safeguarding is a 'mainstream' approach but that Scotland was failing to identify the increased vulnerability of disabled children and their need for additional protection;

» children with communication impairments, behavioural disorders, learning disabilities and sensory impairments are particularly vulnerable;

» England has a range of policies and procedures devoted specifically to safeguarding and improving the lives of disabled children;

» there is a lack of training for professionals and a key area of difficulty is that practitioners lack skills in communicating with disabled children and are poor at recording information;

» some professionals refuse to believe disabled children are abused;

» the sharing of information has greatly improved;

» key people involved with disabled children are often not included in Child Protection Case Conferences; and,

» the justice system fails disabled children.

Stalker et al (2010 highlight Sullivan and Knutson's (2000) large-scale US study of child abuse. It included more than 40,000 children, and concluded that children with disabilities were:

» 3.4 times more likely to be abused than non-disabled children;

» 3.8 times more likely to be neglected and physically abused;

» 3.1 times more likely to be sexually abused; and

» 3.9 times more likely to be emotionally abused.

These frightening statistics showed that 31% of disabled children had been abused, compared with a prevalence rate of 9% among non-disabled children (NSPCC 2003:20). Research also shows that there is an under-reporting of abuse. Mencap's (2007) report, 'Death by Indifference', suggested that only one in 30 cases of sexual abuse of disabled children is reported, compared with one in five of the non-disabled population. Although Sullivan and Knutson's study was undertaken in the USA, several studies have shown similar levels of abuse in the UK. Stalker et al (2010) also suggest that disabled children should receive sex education, safety skills training and information about their rights. A further crucial area they highlight is the need for safeguarding systems to be more considerate towards disabled children and their families, to allow more time for disclosure and the interviewing of disabled children.

When working with children with disabilities and complex health needs, it is important to collaborate with colleagues and other professionals to really understand the child's health and other needs, and to separate the indicators of abuse or harm from the effects of the child's impairment and disability. It is not always immediately evident that a child with a disability has suffered abuse, or what look like signs of abuse may actually be merely a presentation of their condition; for example, a fracture in a child with brittle bone disease (osteogenesis imperfecta). Other indicators of abuse, such as bruising or poor growth, may be attributable to the child's medical condition. It is also essential to consider both non-organic and organic 'failure to thrive' in consultation with colleagues, particularly when considering cases of neglect. You should refer to guidance such as the Department of Health's *Assessing Disabled Children and their Families Practice Guidance* (2000).

It is important to remember that children with disabilities are dependent for medical and personal care and thus have a large number of adults around them on a day-to-day basis to help with eg intimate care such as bathing and toileting. Both the child and their parents may have come to accept this as normal, when in fact it could be demeaning or over-restrictive or, in some circumstances, have become abusive (Clements and Read 2003). This type of dependency may also make the child grow up to believe that others have access to their bodies and they must accept this as the norm. The child may also have a lack of sexual knowledge and a wish to please the person whom they believe is trustworthy, and do not know what is wrong. Some parents or children can be reluctant to report abuse by carers as they may fear that services they depend upon could be withdrawn.

When a child is presenting with challenging behaviour you should consider if this is an indicator of abuse or just related to their condition; for example, a child with autism may have challenging behaviour but you should also consider the demands the parents place on that child and if they are being 'abusive' in their expectations and measures to change the child's behaviour, rather than looking at their own behaviour and changing their responses towards their child. Remember, also, Munro (2011) highlights a tendency to focus on the needs of parents, with insufficient attention given to the needs and concerns of the child. This can be particularly so when working with children with disabilities due to the multiple issues and emotions going on both for the child and parents and/or carer at any one time and the high risk of family breakdown.

DCSF (2009:p 38) states that professionals may find it more difficult to attribute indicators of abuse or neglect, or be reluctant to act on any concerns about a disabled child, due to a number of reasons that they are not 'consciously aware of', such as:

» Over-identifying with the child's parents and carers and being reluctant to accept that abuse or neglect has occurred or is taking place, and instead seeing this as being due to them being stressed because they are caring for a child with disabilities;

» A lack of knowledge about the impact of the disability on the child and what is usual or unusual behaviour for that child, and confusion about those behaviours and the behaviours indicative of a child being abused;

» Not believing that the child's sexualised or self-injurious behaviour is indicative of abuse (this includes denial of the child's sexuality);

» Being unable to communicate with the child or using the wrong method of communication.

It is essential that the worker is not deterred by their concerns not being taken seriously or worries they have 'got it wrong' – the DCSF (2009:p 39) reminds you that '*for some disabled children with speech, language and communication needs, making known that they have been subject to abuse, neglect or ill treatment is dependent on the positive action undertaken by professionals. Thus, it is of the utmost importance that such concerns are passed on.*'

It is very saddening to believe that in today's society the most vulnerable people continue to be more exposed to abuse than their non-disabled peers, despite the robust systems in place designed to protect them.

Research statistics

Contact a Family undertook research on some issues faced by families with disabled children. See the link in 'Taking it further' below for a more in-depth study of this research, but here are just a few findings for you to think about that *may* be contributors to child abuse.

» 52% of families with a disabled child are at risk of experiencing poverty, and 21.8% of families have incomes that are less than half the UK mean. Furthermore, only 16% of mothers with disabled children work, compared with 61% of other mothers.

» It costs up to three times as much to raise a disabled child as it does to raise a child without disabilities.

» Caring for a disabled child can cause relationship problems. Stress, depression and lack of sleep are other commonly experienced problems.

» Pupils with special educational needs (with and without statements) account for 7 in 10 of all permanent exclusions from school. This is the highest rate of permanent exclusions.

» 70% say understanding and acceptance of disability from their community or society is poor ('What Makes my Family Stronger', 2009).

» 50% of families with disabled children say that their isolation is a result of the discrimination or stigma they experience ('Forgotten Families', 2011).

» 96% of parent carers said that their disabled child has been bullied at school ('Bullying of children with disabilities in schools', 2011).

(cited on www.cafamily.org.uk/professionals/research/)

Safeguarding and promoting the welfare of children

Everyone has a duty to safeguard and promote the welfare of children, and child protection is the fundamental basis for intervention and work with children regardless of which area we are working in. When we are talking about safeguarding and promoting the welfare of children the 'Working Together to Safeguard Children' document (DfE 2015:92) defines this as:

» protecting children from maltreatment;

» preventing the impairment of children's health or development;

» ensuring that children are growing up in circumstances consistent with the provision of safe and effective care; and

» taking action to enable all children to have the best life chances.

Sometimes it is difficult, particularly when you may be inexperienced or there are multiple factors to take into consideration, to decide when you cross over into what may be deemed to be a 'child protection' scenario rather than 'child in need' case. It is important to consider what is good enough, what is neglectful and any additional vulnerability factors for each child. This does not mean it is acceptable for a child without a disability to live in neglectful and dirty conditions, but these conditions may have a more severe impact upon a child who, for example, has to be fed by gastrostomy tube or who has other complex health needs and requires clean, sterile conditions. The impact upon the child with a disability could be more significant and may even result in serious illness or death. When making your assessment, you need to think about the risks to the child and what evidence you have that is informing your decisions.

Perhaps this is evidence drawn from your Social Care Assessment, parenting assessments, Child in Need meetings and information from other professionals. You then have to make a judgment about whether you have met the threshold to move to the child protection route. There are strict policies and procedures you must follow once you are making decisions around child protection, such as holding strategy discussions with partner agencies. You should always talk with your manager about any worries and they will support you in your decision making, as they too have to be involved in these procedures. It is usually your manager who would hold the strategy discussion based on the information you provide.

The Children Act 1989 introduced the concept of the 'threshold' for significant harm, and this justifies our decision to take action and undertake statutory intervention in a child's life – in their 'best interests'.

Section 47(1b) of the Children Act 1989 states that:

Where a local authority... have reasonable cause to suspect that a child who lives, or is found, in the area and is suffering, or is likely to suffer, significant harm, the authority shall make such enquiries as they consider necessary to enable them to decide whether they should take any action to safeguard or promote the child's welfare. (DCSF 2010:150)

Let's take a deeper look at what classifies as 'harm'.

What is harm?

Under Section 31(9) of the Children Act 1989, as amended by the Adoption and Children Act 2002 (DCSF 2010:36):

> » harm means ill-treatment or impairment of health or development, including for example impairment suffered by seeing or hearing the ill-treatment of another;
>
> » development means physical, intellectual, emotional, social or behavioural development;
>
> » health means physical or mental health;
>
> » ill-treatment includes sexual abuse and forms of ill-treatment that are not physical.

The Adoption and Children Act 2002 has since broadened the definition of significant harm to include the emotional harm suffered by children 'seeing or hearing the ill treatment of another', ie they may witness domestic violence or are aware of domestic violence within their home environment. The legislation recognises this affects the child even though they may not actually see what is happening (see www.legislation. gov.uk/ukpga/2002/38/section/120).

There are no absolute criteria on which to rely when you are making your judgment as to what constitutes significant harm, but you should give consideration to the severity of ill-treatment. It may be one single traumatic event or it may be a succession of significant events, both 'acute and long-standing, which interrupt, change or damage the child's physical, social and psychological development. Long-term physical or emotional abuse can cause impairment to such an extent that it constitutes significant harm' (DCSF 2008b:p 81). Factors in significant harm may include:

- The degree/nature and extent of physical harm, including threats and coercion
- The child's development and disability – their development within their environment and wider family environment (think of the assessment framework)
- The duration and frequency of abuse or neglect
- The extent of premeditation and planning by the perpetrator
- Any additional needs such as medical conditions or disabilities that may affect the child's development and the care they are receiving
- Evidence of sadism or bizarre/unusual elements in child sexual abuse

(DCSF 2010:36–37)

Under Section 31(10) of the Children Act 1989:

Where the question of whether harm suffered by a child is significant turns on the child's health and development, his health or development shall be compared with that which could reasonably be expected of a similar child.

Before we move on to look at an activity about child abuse (harm), we will quickly look at the categories of abuse according to 'Working Together 2015' (DfE 2015:92–93).

Categories of abuse

Sexual abuse

Involves forcing or enticing a child or young person to take part in sexual activities, not necessarily involving a high level of violence, whether or not the child is aware of what is happening. The activities may involve physical contact, including assault by penetration (for example, rape or oral sex) or non-penetrative acts such as masturbation, kissing, rubbing and touching outside of clothing. They may also include non-contact activities, such as involving children in looking at, or in the production of, sexual images, watching sexual activities, encouraging children to behave in sexually inappropriate ways, or grooming a child in preparation for abuse (including via the

Internet). Sexual abuse is not solely perpetrated by adult males. Women can also commit acts of sexual abuse, as can other children.

Grooming

Sexual abuse includes 'grooming a child in preparation for abuse' and it is important to think about what 'grooming' means. When sexual offenders are considering sexually abusing children the grooming process is calculated, and can include grooming both parent and child and other trusted adults who are around the child. Grooming involves gaining the confidence and trust of the child, and those who protect and care for them, in order for the abuser to be able to carry out their abuse. When working with children with a disability consider that they are already vulnerable in many ways – this may be due to their lack of understanding, a communication impairment or having multiple carers undertaking their personal care needs. Another consideration may be that their carer/ parent is vulnerable to abuse, perhaps due to stress, isolation resulting in low self-esteem or tiredness from caring for a child with complex health needs, and therefore can also be a target for grooming. It is well known that people who abuse children unfortunately do not 'stand out'– they are often in positions of power or trust and will work hard to prevent colleagues and friends from having any suspicion that they are abusing children. They befriend vulnerable families to get access to the child, often making themselves indispensable to the parent by helping care for the child. Their friends and the wider community see the abuser as a good character, always offering a 'helping hand' and giving the parent a 'well-deserved break' and thus the abuser gains their trust and takes away suspicion. While we are certainly not saying that you should be suspicious of everyone, you need to be aware that children with disabilities are at a higher risk of abuse simply because of their additional vulnerabilities.

You should also remember that children with disabilities can be vulnerable at home in their bedroom playing on their computer or Xbox, as they can be a target for Internet or cyber bullying by abusers who pretend to be a child and befriend them online.

We suggest that you do further reading on grooming and the 'cycle of abuse'. The National Society for the Prevention of Cruelty to Children (NSPCC) website has lots of useful information about these issues, and the National Crime Agency's Child Exploitation and Online Protection safety centre website (NCA CEOP) is a great resource for safeguarding children from online abuse (see 'Taking it further' at the end of this chapter for links).

A note: Talking about sex and relationships

All children should always be protected from sexual harm and pornography, however, it is important to remember that children are exposed to sexual images and discussions about sexual issues on a daily basis, even when parents are protective and observe the watershed on television. Children still hear about sexual assault, see naked images on the news or watch ongoing television dramas that include discussions of a sexual nature. It is important not to ignore the fact that all children see these things and will be aware of sex to some extent. Therefore, we should not think that just because a child has a disability they won't understand much of what they are hearing, or if they are not able to understand, that they are not still seeing such images.

Activity: **Sexual issues**

Some young people with disabilities go on to have consensual sexual relationships as they mature into adulthood, and therefore it is even more important that they are supported, given appropriate information and knowledge about sexual health and relationships and that they are able to ask questions about sex. This can be difficult for many parents to accept as they have to acknowledge their disabled child as a 'sexual being' with rights to have sex and relationships and to make decisions about their own sexuality. For those young people with more complex disabilities who may not be able to enter into physical sexual relationships, it does not mean that they will not have the same sexual drives and feelings as their non-disabled peers. Their bodies are still developing, with 'raging' hormones and puberty as they enter adolescence even if they may cognitively not be meeting the same developmental milestones or have any understanding of what is happening to their bodies. Therefore, they may still be acting out sexual behaviour but not know how to control these feelings and emotions, thus exposing themselves to more risk. It is important that parents and carers and those professionals working with children with disabilities do not ignore sexual issues, and understand that children have sexual feelings that they need to be able to express safely and appropriately.

What makes some children more vulnerable to sexual abuse than others?

Take a few minutes to think about what makes children with disabilities more vulnerable to sexual abuse than other children.

Think about issues such as:

» the child's cognitive age and their 'actual' developmental stage – this may have been impaired due to their disability;

» multiple carers involved in their day-to-day care – why might this be an issue? child development – what does that tell you about a child's beliefs, ie how they trust adults because we always say, 'If in danger talk to a policeman, or your teacher' etc;

» they might not be able to differentiate between the motives of those who are caring for them and those who may want to harm them;

» the child's sexual curiosity – child development and sexual maturity.

Also, what do we actually tell children about sex and sexuality and keeping safe? What do we tell a child with a disability about sex? Probably in reality, not a lot. Should a disabled young adult even have sex? People will have different views about this regardless of the young person's own rights and desires. Think about media and the availability of sexual images and pornographic material.

How can you help protect children and young people from harm but at the same time encourage their natural curiosity at a level that is appropriate to their own 'age and stage' of development and their disability?

Neglect

The persistent failure to meet a child's basic physical and/or psychological needs, likely to result in the serious impairment of the child's health or development. Neglect may occur during pregnancy as a result of maternal substance abuse. Once a child is born, neglect may involve a parent or carer failing to provide adequate food, clothing and shelter, including exclusion from home or abandonment; failure to protect a child from physical and emotional harm or danger; failing to ensure adequate supervision (including the use of inadequate care-givers); or failing to ensure access to appropriate medical care or treatment. It may also include neglect of, or unresponsiveness to, a child's basic emotional needs. (DfE 2015:93)

It is important to remember that neglect can *fluctuate* in both level and duration and can improve with services but then deteriorate again after they are withdrawn because progress has been made. When determining the next steps in neglect cases the decisions need to be both timely and decisive in order that children are not left in neglectful conditions (DfE 2015:26). It is also important therefore to consider if services need to be put in place during the assessment rather than waiting until it has been completed. You also need to ensure, however, that you consider 'good enough' parenting and that services are not put in place 'just in case'.

Parents who are caring for children with complex health needs and disabilities are by definition more likely to be exhausted than those parents caring for non-disabled children and you must consider within your assessments the physical and emotional demands, time constraints and additional day-to-day pressures upon parents with children with disabilities. Although you should not lower your expectations for those parents and the care their child should receive, you should consider the additional pressure and stress that some parents may be managing and the additional support they may require as a result of these pressures.

Emotional abuse (or psychological abuse)

This category has evolved over recent years to include changes in the world to reflect technological and social developments, and now includes abuse over the Internet (cyber bullying). Emotional abuse is:

The persistent emotional maltreatment of a child such as to cause severe and persistent adverse effects on the child's emotional development. It may involve conveying to a child that they are worthless or unloved, inadequate, or valued only insofar as they meet the needs of another person. It may include not giving the child opportunities to express their views, deliberately silencing them or 'making fun' of what they say or how they communicate. It may feature age or developmentally inappropriate expectations being imposed on children. These may include interactions that are beyond a child's developmental capability, as well as overprotection and limitation of exploration and learning, or preventing the child participating in normal social interaction. It may involve seeing or hearing the ill-treatment of another. It may involve serious bullying (including cyber bullying), causing children frequently to feel frightened or in danger, or the exploitation or corruption of children. Some level of emotional abuse is involved in all types of maltreatment of a child, though it may occur alone. (DfE 2015:92–93)

Physical abuse

May include '*hitting, shaking, throwing, poisoning, burning or scalding, drowning, suffocating or otherwise causing physical harm to a child. Physical harm may also be caused when a parent or carer* fabricates *the symptoms of, or deliberately induces, illness in a child.*' (DfE 2015:92)

See Chapter 11 'Taking it further' for an activity that considers possible abusive scenarios.

Fabricated illness (or induced illness)

The terminology around fabricated illness has been debated and changed over the years. It was commonly known as Munchausen's syndrome by proxy, factitious illness by proxy or illness induction syndrome, and the terminology is used by some as if it were a psychiatric diagnosis (DCSF 2008b:2). We focus here not on the name of the condition used but the impact of the fabricated or induced illness upon the child's health and development, and how best to safeguard and promote the child's welfare.

There are three main ways of fabricating or inducing illness in a child (these are not mutually exclusive), including:

> » *fabrication* of signs and symptoms. This may include fabrication of past medical history;

> » fabrication of signs and symptoms and *falsification* of hospital charts and records, or even specimens of bodily fluids. This may also include falsification of letters and documents;

> » *induction* of illness by a variety of means.

You should consider what is being reported by the parent or carer and how the child is presenting, but do not jump to conclusions: you need to make a distinction between parents who are very anxious because their child is poorly and those who are displaying abnormal behaviour. Some parents may panic and not know what is normal for their child, for example if their child is newly diagnosed with an illness; they may present as over-anxious and repeatedly present at hospital requesting various investigations or medical treatments. In these cases you could use a multi-agency approach with the support of skilled professionals such as Learning Disability Community Nurses, to help parents learn how to interpret their child's health needs, how to manage the child's condition and know what is usual for their child. Health professionals should familiarise themselves with the various presentations of this type of child abuse. In these circumstances, they should consider whether any child is having their health or development impaired (DCSF 2008b:para 3.10).

Concerns may arise about possible fabricated or induced illness when:

> » reported symptoms and signs found on examination are not explained by any medical condition from which the child may be suffering;

> » physical examination and results of medical investigations do not explain reported symptoms and signs;

» there is an inexplicably poor response to prescribed medication and other treatment;

» new symptoms are reported on resolution of previous ones;

» reported symptoms and found signs are not seen to begin in the absence of the carer;

» over time the child is repeatedly presented with a range of signs and symptoms;

» the child's normal, daily life activities are being curtailed, for example school attendance, beyond that which might be expected for any medical disorder from which the child is known to suffer (DCSF 2008b:para 4.5).

Such abnormal behaviour can be present in one or more carers and often involves the passive compliance of the child. These carer behaviours may constitute ill-treatment (Section 31(9) of the Children Act 1989) and where the parents' presentation or child's impairment is such that there are concerns the child is suffering or is likely to suffer significant harm, 'Safeguarding children in whom illness is fabricated or induced (2008c)' should be consulted in line with your organisation's safeguarding policies and procedures.

(www.gov.uk/government/uploads/system/uploads/attachment_data/file/277314/Safeguarding_Children_in_whom_illness_is_fabricated_or_induced.pdf)

Any concerns need to be discussed with those health professionals involved with the child, including their GP. When working with children with disabilities it is important to consider that there may be multiple professionals involved with the child, including occupational therapists, speech and language therapists, specialist nurse practitioners, several paediatricians if the child has multiple conditions and/or has specialists at different hospitals, teachers and teaching assistants, hospice staff and care assistants. Thus a co-ordinated and 'joined up' approach is required at all times and not just when there may be a concern or worry about a child.

Case study: Piecing things together

Joanne is the mother of six-year-old Timmy. Mark is Timmy's father: he works abroad and is home for one week out of every four weeks. When Mark is at home he gives lots of attention and time to Timmy, to make up for the time he is not there. Timmy has presented with severe vomiting at school and at home, and there is an assessment being undertaken by social worker Jenny as

Joanne has requested support or respite as she feels that the vomiting is getting difficult to manage, and that there is no support for her when Mark is away. Jenny has visited Timmy's school, who are worried that they have been unable to find out the cause of the vomiting; the school nurse has been monitoring Timmy's diet to explore allergies or intolerances, but they have been unable to find any patterns or types of food that trigger it. A consultant paediatrician has been involved for two years as Timmy had previously attended A&E and health records show some queries around projectile vomiting or intolerances to dairy, gluten, lactose etc. Various tests had been carried out, but nothing was identified as a certain cause. At school Timmy is presenting as wan and tired, and has recently lost weight: measuring against previous routine checks shows that there has been a significant weight loss but at a very gradual rate, so it had gone unnoticed until Timmy's skin was noted to be quite pale and his eyes drawn, with dark circles. School report to Jenny that there has been good communication with Joanne, who has informed of his vomiting through the night and suggested how tired he might be. Joanne is reported to keep school well informed of recent appointments and tests, and feels that she is managing the situation as best she can; however, she is looking tired and drawn herself, and agreed with her need for support. School feel that Joanne is a very positive person who will volunteer in school to help Timmy's class with reading and snack times etc even though she has a lot on herself.

As part of the assessment Jenny pulls together information as it had been noted that the chronology of the case so far was brief and that there were gaps which needed to be filled to show a full picture. In completing and filling in the gaps in the chronology, Jenny identified a pattern in that Timmy's vomiting occurred daily for a few weeks at a time, but then there were gaps when he was not vomiting for a whole week at a time.

What do you think the chronology is telling you? What patterns are showing?

Suggestions: The weeks of no vomiting are tying in with Mark being home? The vomiting is only occurring when Joanne has care for Timmy on her own?

What other information might you need to help you understand more about what might be happening?

Suggestions: Explore the hospital visits to see if they tie in with Joanne being on her own. Does Timmy stay with other family members, and if so, what happens there?

Gather more detail from the school about when the vomiting happens: is it in the mornings or at other times of the day?

Gather more information from Joanne around what her worries are about Timmy's vomiting, when it started etc. What was happening around the family at this time? Any emotional trauma or upset, depression, Mark starting a new job etc?

See link in 'Taking it further' to read more about the importance of chronologies, building a fuller picture and patterns of behaviours or situations that can show what is happening in a child's life. It also details a real case of fabricated illness that resulted in a mother being convicted, and gives a list of tips on how to approach with caution.

Prevent agenda

The Prevent Strategy (2011) is part of the UK government's wider counter-terrorism strategy, CONTEST, which came about after the 2005 London bombings and has continued following subsequent worldwide atrocities, security threats and major incidents, and the rising fears about people being drawn into 'radicalisation'.

Section 26 of the Counter-Terrorism and Security Act 2015 places a duty on certain bodies (this includes the police, prisons, probation service, National Health Service, educational establishments and local authorities) in the exercise of their functions, to have 'due regard to the need to prevent people from being drawn into terrorism'. This statutory guidance is issued under Section 29 of the Counter-Terrorism and Security Act 2015. The Act states that the authorities subject to the provisions must have regard to this guidance when carrying out their duties (HM Gov 2015:3). The four strategies under the Act are to Pursue, Prepare, Protect and Prevent.

Prevent aims to identify vulnerable people, including those young people or adults with learning disabilities, who are at risk of being targeted by extremists and may become radicalised, and to work with those who are either being targeted or may be thought to be responding to extremism and the ideology of terrorism (HM Gov 2015).

See 'Taking it further' again for a link to a great briefing note from the Home Office and Department for Education aimed at head teachers, teachers and safeguarding leads that provides advice about online terrorist and extreme material. It includes a short summary of some of the main ISIS (Islamic State of Iraq and Syria) propaganda claims and identifies social media sites ISIS is using.

Female genital mutilation

Female genital mutilation or FGM is illegal in the UK but is more common than most people realise, both in the UK and worldwide. FGM is a collective term for procedures that include the removal of part or all of the external female genitalia, done for cultural or other 'non-therapeutic' reasons. FGM is sometimes performed on newborn infants, but is more often carried out on girls between the ages of 4–15 (ie before puberty); it may also on occasions be performed on women before pregnancy or marriage (DCSF 2010:195).

What happens when someone is concerned about a child?

If at any time it is considered that the child may be a child in need as defined in the Children Act 1989, or that the child has suffered significant harm or is likely to do so, a referral should be made immediately to local authority children's social care. This referral can be made by any professional. (DfE 2015:14)

Anyone can make a referral if they have any concerns about a child. If the person is aware that the child already has a social worker it is usual to contact that social worker directly to discuss their worries. If the worker is not available, there would usually be a duty social worker they can speak to. If you/they are really worried about the child, or they do not have a social worker, don't delay and telephone the local authority customer service team (this may be called a Multi-Agency Safeguarding Hub – MASH), who will be able to either redirect you to the appropriate person or team, or take the details directly. If you have concerns out of normal office hours you should ring the local authority Emergency Duty Team (and/or police if felt necessary because of worries about immediate harm).

Once contact has been made a decision will be made within one working day on whether to proceed to a referral and look at what are the most appropriate next steps. Some options are:

» No further action (nfa)

» Advice and information given

» Consideration to direct to other agencies or 'early help' support (such as Early Help Assessment, Team Around the Child, family support etc)

» Proceed under Section 17 Child in Need procedures*

» Proceed under Section 47 Child Protection procedures*

(*involves a Social Care Assessment being completed by a social worker under the Framework for the Assessment of Children in Need and Their Families 2000)

The procedures are the same for a child with a disability as they are for a non-disabled child. The decision will be made with consideration to what evidence is presented at the time the contact is made, what impairment there may be to the child's health or development, and if the child is suffering or likely to suffer significant harm that justifies an assessment to establish whether the child is in need. The decision will normally be made following discussions with the referring professionals/service, the review of any information already held on file, and collaboration with other services as required, including the police if a criminal offence may have taken place (DCSF 2010).

Emergency protection orders

There may be occasions when there is an IMMEDIATE risk to the life of a child or a risk of immediate harm, and in those situations the police, local authority social workers or NSPCC are able to use their statutory child protection powers that allow them to *act immediately to secure the safety of a child*. When it is felt that the child must be removed from their home, the local authority must, wherever possible and unless a child's safety is otherwise at immediate risk, apply for an Emergency Protection Order (EPO) (DfE 2015:31).

There are circumstances when a court may include an exclusion requirement in an EPO or an interim care order (s38A and s44A of the Children Act 1989). This allows a perpetrator to be removed from the home instead of having to remove the child (DfES 2006:52).

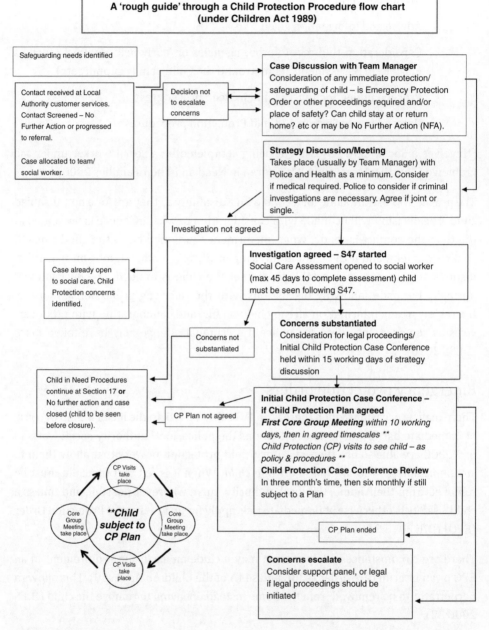

Figure 2.1 Concern for a child under Section 47 child protection procedures (adapted from DfE 2015 pp 38 and 48)

Strategy Meetings/Discussions

Children's Services must hold a Strategy Meeting whenever there is reasonable cause to suspect that a child has suffered or is likely to suffer significant harm, regardless of whether it appears that a criminal offence against a child has been committed. Where a meeting cannot be held, a Strategy Discussion may be held (between the Team Manager (or equivalent) and the police/health services) over the telephone usually due to the urgency and geographical locations of other professionals. A series of telephone discussions may be required. The purpose of the Strategy Meeting (or discussion) is to decide whether a Section 47 enquiry under the Children Act 1989 is required and if so, to develop a plan of action for the Section 47 enquiry between agencies.

The Strategy Meeting should involve, as a *minimum*, Children's Services, the police, health professionals and the referring agency. Other agencies involved with the family should be included as appropriate, ie school/nursery setting, housing, substance misuse teams or mental health services. For children with disabilities, where possible and when time allows, a planned pre-arranged meeting is much better than a strategy discussion in order to ensure that all necessary professionals are available to contribute to the meeting. This is due in part to the additional complexities associated with many disabilities, for example health issues that affect the child. There may be other issues that have to be discussed if considering removing a child to a safe place, such as trained carers being required to manage the care regime for the child or specialist moving and handling equipment being required. Parents/carers are not invited to a strategy meeting, but the attendants should ensure that the discussion identifies what information will be shared with the child and family. You need to ask yourself, 'If I share this information would this place a child at risk of significant harm or jeopardise police investigations?' – but you need to balance this against their right to be informed (DfE 2015:37). You may wish to invite a representative from your local authority's legal department if it is felt necessary.

Initial Child Protection Case Conference (ICPCC)

The purpose of an Initial Child Protection Case Conference is to bring together all relevant professionals that are involved with the child and family, the parent/carers, supporters and advocates, and where appropriate the child, to analyse, in an inter-agency setting, all relevant information and plan how best to safeguard and promote the welfare of the child. It is the responsibility of the conference to make recommendations on how agencies work together to safeguard the child in future, and having decided that the criteria are met, the chair of the conference must ensure that the category of abuse is determined. From their assessment the social worker would have to present the information about the reason for the conference, their understanding of the child's needs, parental capacity and family and environmental context, and evidence of how the child has been abused or neglected and its impact on their health and development (DfE 2015:43).

Review conferences should be held within three months of the ICPCC and then at least every six months while the plan is in place. Reviews are held to check the safety, health and development of the child against the planned outcomes set out in the child protection plan (CPP); ensure that the child continues to be safeguarded from harm; and consider whether the CPP should continue to be in place or should be changed (DfE 2015).

Independent Reviewing Officer (IRO)

It is the role of the IRO to ensure that a child's care planning and review process is being effectively managed. An IRO would chair review meetings such as:

» ICPCCs and Review Child Protection Case Conferences; and

» Looked-After Children's Reviews – including those for children subject to Care Orders and those looked after under Section 20 and Section 20 Regulation 48 short breaks (See Chapter 1).

An IRO should be able to offer an independent oversight of a child's case to ensure that the child's interests are kept at the forefront of the decision making. The IRO must speak to the child in private prior to the review to ensure they have understood the child's wishes and feelings and established that they are aware of the decisions that are being made for them and why. An IRO should also consider the child's right to have an advocate. There are obvious difficulties, as we have discussed throughout this book, when communicating with some children and young people who have severe and profound disabilities, including communication difficulties; however the IRO should make efforts to communicate effectively with the child, with specialist support should this be required. Consideration should also be given as to how information is fed back to the child after the meeting (DCSF 2010c).

Child Protection Plans

When a child has been made the subject of a plan, the outline CPP is prepared by the child protection conference, together with the core group members, based on the findings of the assessment and contributions from reports, professionals, family members and any other evidence presented at the meeting. This plan should follow the dimensions relating to a child's developmental needs, parenting capacity and family and environmental factors, and draw on knowledge about effective interventions across agencies and age ranges. It should:

» Ensure the child is safe from harm and prevent the child from suffering further harm;

» Promote the child's health and development and show clearly what needs to change, by how much, and by when in order for the child to be safe and have their needs met;

» Support immediate and wider family members to safeguard and promote the welfare of their child, provided it is in the best interests of the child (DfE 2015:45).

Core groups

When a child has been made the subject of a CPP, the conference decides the membership of a core group of practitioners and family members who develop and implement the CPP that was prepared at the ICPCC. The core group then meet within 10 working days of the ICPCC and continue to meet sufficiently frequently to monitor the plan and its outcomes while a child remains subject to it. As discussed above, there may be large numbers of professionals involved who attend an ICPCC (or CIN Meetings). When considering which professionals need to be part of the core group meetings, it may be that these numbers are reduced to 'key' professionals, and that only one or two health professionals attend who can then liaise and feedback to their colleagues in order to keep the core groups manageable and not too daunting for the child and family. All the professionals who attended the ICPCC, however, would usually attend the Child Protection Case Conference Review (CPCCR).

The lead social worker must be an employee of a 'statutory body' (Children's Social Care or the NSPCC) and should be qualified and experienced (DfE 2015). The core group takes joint responsibility for developing the CPP as a detailed working tool, and implementing it, based on the outline plan agreed at the ICPCC and subsequent reviews. The child should be included where they have age and understanding and should be encouraged to contribute throughout the process. Often you may find that some children with disabilities will not be able to understand the process, but this does not mean that their wishes and feelings should not be explored and shared at each meeting (see Chapter 4). The child's best interests should always remain paramount.

Child protection visits

A child subject to a CPP must be seen by the social worker and each Local Safeguarding Children's Board (LSCB) will have policies and procedures for when the child should be seen, depending upon the severity of the risks involved. The frequency of contact should be stipulated in the CPP, and this should include seeing the child alone, seeing a baby awake on some visits and visiting the child's bedroom. If a parent or carer is avoiding this or refusing to let the child be seen, it must be viewed as a serious breach of the CPP and you should always discuss this with your manager. It is usual practice to also undertake unannounced visits.

The visits should include undertaking any direct work with the child and family in accordance with the CPP, taking into account the child's wishes and feelings and the views of the parents in so far as they are consistent with the child's welfare (DfE 2015:45). Eileen Munro, in her final report, reminds us that *'it is crucial that the child is seen (alone when appropriate) by the lead social worker in accordance with the CP Plan: the child should be spoken and listened to and their wishes and feelings ascertained (in accordance with their age and understanding).'* (Munroe 2011:150)

It is worth remembering that despite the intervention, monitoring or further assessment that you undertake either while in the child protection arena (or CIN procedures), you may reach the conclusion that the situation is not safe and the child needs to be removed in order to protect them from harm. You should never make this decision in isolation and should consult your manager as well as take legal advice from your local authority's solicitors.

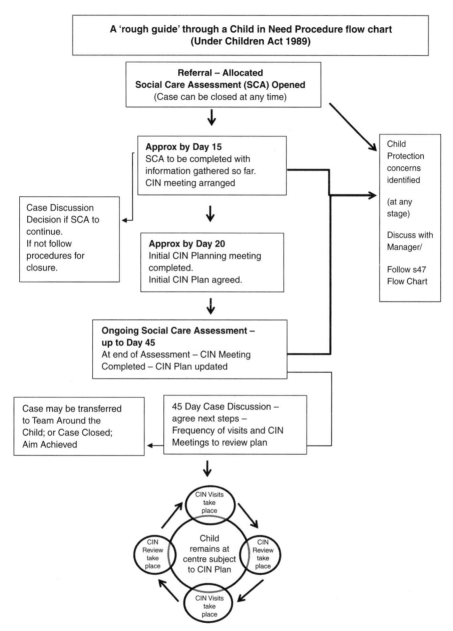

Figure 2.2 Referral of a child following the Section 17 Child in Need process (adapted from DfE 2015 p 35)

Child in Need explained

When you are working with a child and family under Section 17 of the Children Act 1989 you need to bear in mind that this is voluntary involvement by the family and they can choose to end the involvement of social care at any time.

A child in need is defined under the Children Act 1989 as a child who is unlikely to achieve or maintain a reasonable level of health or development, or whose health and development is likely to be significantly or further impaired, without the provision of services; or a child who is disabled. Children in need may be assessed under Section 17 of the Children Act 1989, in relation to their special educational needs, disabilities, as a carer, or because they have committed a crime. Where an assessment takes place, it will be carried out by a social worker. (DfE 2015:18)

Whilst working with children under Section 17, CIN, you should always monitor the situation carefully over time, to ensure that the child remains safeguarded, by working with other professionals who are involved with the child and in consultation with the child and their family. If you believe children to be at risk of harm and you feel the worries are too high to remain at Section 17, you should discuss your concerns with your manager about 'next steps', or if this requires further action either by implementing other interventions and strategies under Section 17, or instigating child protection procedures if it is deemed necessary. It is essential that you are having regular case supervision with your manager and 'case discussions' as the case progresses, and that these are recorded clearly on file showing how decisions were made. The social work manager should challenge the social worker's assumptions, and these processes allow an informed decision to be taken regarding the nature of any action required and which services should be provided. There are often multiple professionals involved with the child with disabilities but you may also be working with relevant professionals that are involved with the parent/carer if they have identified additional needs, for example the parent may have a learning difficulty or mental health problems and have an adult social care social worker or community psychiatric nurse or both. The police may also be involved if there are concerns about domestic violence, or if a parent is in prison the probation service may need to participate. Housing may also be involved regarding any necessary adaptations.

Scenario: Look who is working with Eddie

Eddie was a four-year-old, non-disabled boy who had just started at his local school in the Reception class. Having just come home from school Eddie was asked by his mum to go upstairs and change out of his uniform. While Eddie's mother was in the kitchen washing dishes and preparing tea she did not hear Eddie open the front door. He went into the garden and saw his older brother's friend playing across the road. Eddie went to see the boy, stepped into the road and was run over by a taxi. The taxi driver did not stop. Eddie was seriously injured and was airlifted to the local hospital where he had to undergo a life-saving operation and subsequent operations. He was in hospital for five months and was left with permanent and substantial disabilities. Eddie's and his family's lives were never the same again. After an initial safeguarding investigation under Section 47 it was deemed that there was no further action needed under safeguarding procedures and Eddie's case was managed under Section 17, Child in Need. Eddie's mother and close family had to receive training to meet Eddie's health needs. The diagram below shows the professionals and family members who attended the CIN meetings over the first 12 months of Eddie's case being opened by the social worker managing his case as a 'child in need'.

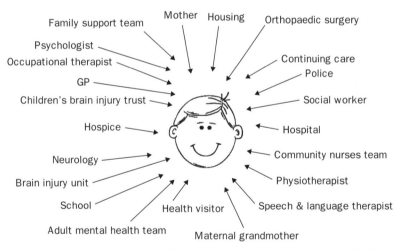

Figure 2.3 Professionals and family members who attend the Child in Need meetings

You must not think that if you are working with children at CIN level that you are not managing risk. Risk is always prevalent with every case, particularly with children with disabilities. You should consider the disability and balance risks to a child. When a case is managed at CIN level there should be regular CIN meetings and the child should be seen on a regular basis, usually in different settings (but this should always include seeing the child at home), and timescales should again be discussed and agreed with your manager and recorded within supervision notes. The child must also have a CIN Plan.

Child in Need Meetings/Reviews

CIN Reviews should involve all relevant professionals involved with the child, and where appropriate those involved with the parents (as discussed above). The parents and child (where appropriate) must attend all meetings. The purpose of the meeting is to agree and make changes to the CIN Plan as the case develops.

Child in Need Plans

A CIN Plan is drawn up following a Social Care Assessment that identifies the child's needs and where a coordinated response is necessary to meet those needs. When you are completing a CIN Plan you should include:

» the identified developmental needs of the child

» any services required to meet the identified assessed need

» timescales required for actions

» specific, achievable, child-focused outcomes intended to promote and safeguard the welfare of the child.

(See Chapter 11 'Taking it further' for an example of a CIN Plan for Olivia, who we discuss below.)

Managing complex cases

Ordinarily we would be very concerned to hear about a child being locked in their bedroom and would most likely consider this as an issue for child protection and safeguarding for many reasons, such as restriction of the child's liberty, concerns of abuse and neglect and risks of fire and other safety issues etc. There are occasions, however, when it has been agreed to use a lock on a door, as a last resort when absolutely necessary and subject to regular reviews and continued assessment.

Here we look at Olivia's case that was held at CIN Section 17, where Olivia was locked in her bedroom at night. The social worker completed the following Joint Agency Risk to Safety Assessment Agreement, which was agreed and signed by all the professionals at Olivia's CIN Meeting. The risks are self-explanatory.

Scenario: To lock or not to lock? Example 1

On 11 January 2016 a referral was made by Dr Fixer, Consultant Community Paediatrician. Dr Fixer requested a Social Care Assessment for overnight respite care for Olivia because he was worried that her parents were exhausted and at their wits' end due to her behaviour. The assessment was completed on 5 March 2016. Olivia was observed at school by Eric Helper, CAMHS, who noted behavioural difficulties such as hitting, spitting, screeching and urinating. Parents reported Olivia has tried to drink bleach and other household liquids, light the gas oven, and reached for knives or other sharp objects; she requires supervision at all times. During the assessment being completed it was highlighted that Olivia was locked in her bedroom at night, therefore as part of the CIN Plan it has been identified that a risk to safety assessment agreement is to be completed in order to make a decision about the appropriateness of locking Olivia's door. (Her bedroom could not be moved to another area in the house.)

What is the risk to be assessed?

1. *Olivia being locked in her bedroom at night and the fire risk that this poses.*

2. *Door in kitchen not being fireproof.*

3. *Positioning of Olivia's bedroom off the kitchen, resulting in the accessibility being limited should there be a fire.*

4. *Olivia's behaviour, autism and disability.*

Who is the risk to?

1. *Olivia.*

2. *Family members should there be a fire and them intervening.*

What has been done to minimise the risk?

1. Olivia being locked in her bedroom at night and fire risk:

   » *Star lock outside the bedroom door, so there is always a key to be able to access the room.*

   » *Kitchen door and dining room doors are always closed at night; however, they are not fire doors.*

> » *Back door key is left by the front door; however, discussions to be held about having a key always in a key safe outside the property, should they not be able to access the one near the front door.*
>
> » *While in her bedroom, wardrobes are securely fastened to the walls; wardrobe doors are locked; bedroom window ledge is sloping to prevent climbing; window has a restrictor and a lock which are always secured; and there is a baby monitor (sound not camera) locked in her wardrobe so that when she does wake parents are able to hear straight away.*
>
> » *Mrs Green sits outside Olivia's bedroom until she is asleep.*
>
> » *Bathroom door is locked and shut.*
>
> » *The bed is secure and heavy so Olivia cannot lift this off the floor.*
>
> » *All liquids and sharp objects to be stored in a lockable cupboard. Gas oven replaced by electric oven*
>
> » *At night there are two adults in the property to support each other.*
>
> » *There are three smoke alarms in the property.*
>
> » *A joint visit has been completed with Milly Maxi, occupational therapist, and the risks have been highlighted and shared.*

2. Door in kitchen not being fireproof:

> » *Fire service will be contacted to complete home visit and provide any recommendations.*
>
> » *Housing to be contacted to share the risk and highlight the worries regarding the door not being fireproof.*
>
> » *Family always making sure that the door is closed at night to delay as much as possible any spread of fire.*

3. Positioning of Olivia's bedroom off the kitchen, resulting in the accessibility being limited should there be a fire:

> » *Fire service to complete a fire escape plan with the family.*
>
> » *Key to be in a key safe to ensure that they will be able to access a key at all times.*

» *Dining room and kitchen doors to be fireproof as this would provide more time to get to Olivia.*

» *There is a hallway between the dining room/kitchen and Olivia's bedroom with doors either side providing access to the garden.*

4. Olivia's behaviour, autism and disabilities:

» *CAMHS are involved and supporting the family.*

» *School are very supportive and offer advice and behaviour strategies.*

» *The bedroom door is locked because in the past Olivia has gained access to the kitchen and lit the oven rings; smashed glasses and cut herself; emptied cupboards; and put any item/substance in her mouth, such as knives and bleach. Olivia does not have an understanding of danger and should she have access to the rest of the property she would be at risk of significant harm and also place other family members at risk.*

» *Social Care providing Short Breaks and Direct Payments.*

How will this risk be monitored and by whom:

All of the risks will be shared within the CIN meeting, which is being held on 30 March, and a copy of the risk assessment will be shared and signed by parents and all professionals and this will be reviewed at future CIN meetings.

Future actions:

1. *Social worker to contact fire service for them to assess the property, share the risk and make them aware that Olivia is in the property and locked in the bedroom at night.*

2. *Parents test smoke alarms once a week to ensure that these are working and change if not.*

3. *Parents to purchase a key safe to be fitted.*

4. *Fire safety tools eg fire blanket and extinguisher to be purchased by parents if not supplied by fire service.*

5. *All liquids/hazardous substances and knives to be placed in lockable cupboard and gas cooker to be changed for electric cooker.*

Agreed and signed by:

Jenni Jinks, Social Worker:	*Team Manager:*
Mr Green:	*Mrs Green:*
Eric Helper, CAMHS:	*Irene Learner, Teacher:*
Ivor Waters, fire service:	*Milly Maxi, OT:*
Dr Fixer, paediatrician:	

A lock being used is often only agreed following the completion of a risk assessment, and in the authors' experience the risk assessment would be completed using a multi-disciplinary approach. A meeting should take place with key professionals, for example, OTs, other health professionals and community nurses, social worker, CAMHS and parents. Furthermore, a risk assessment would not usually be agreed until a fire safety check had been undertaken by the local fire brigade, with an agreed safety plan being put in place so that the family have an escape plan to follow in an emergency. The fire officers would also usually ensure that they have a note in their records that there is a vulnerable person living at the address and that there is a locked door. Only then would it be that the risk assessment was agreed and signed by all parties. It is only agreed as a last resort and when the child is at a lower risk being in a room that has a lock on the outside than being allowed access to other areas of the home. It would be expected that other options are explored first, as in the above example.

Here is an example, for comparison, where it was deemed that it was *not* appropriate for a lock to be used:

Scenario: To lock or not to lock? Example 2

William is four years old and lives with his parents Emma and Gary and his younger brother Callum, aged three. William has been diagnosed with severe autism, global developmental delay and pica (this is an appetite for substances that are largely non-nutritive, such as paper, metal, chalk, soil, glass or sand). It is also believed that William has ADHD but due to his age he has not yet been formally diagnosed. He attends full time at Learn Better School. William is non-verbal and communicates through some limited eye contact, noises, smiles and cries. His general wishes and feelings are therefore assumed through observations of his interactions with others and his surroundings and his behaviour with those who know him best.

William is constantly on the go and is always searching for food due to his pica. He has no concept of danger and will climb on anything he can to try to obtain food. William displays some difficult behaviours, including headbutting, biting, pulling hair and kicking, although it is not felt that he intends to hurt anyone. William smears and will try to eat it and make himself sick by regurgitating. He is a poor sleeper despite being on medication, only sleeping for a few broken hours each night. Parents had previously been locking William in a tent during the night to ensure his safety, which raised concerns during an assessment. It could be viewed as a safeguarding concern and it was vital that as part of the assessment the social worker understood the reasons for this. Through further investigation and discussion, it became apparent that his parents felt they had no other way of maintaining William's safety during the night: if he could roam about at night he may climb out of the window, eat his carpet, ingest the paint on his radiator or fall down the stairs due to his limited depth perception – in effect throw himself down the stairs. This was explored with the parents and it was explained that in no circumstance was the padlocking of a tent appropriate.

Suggestions were made to the family and support offered in respect of a parent staying in William's room during the night to monitor him, with support provided to them in the day so they could rest. Despite a level of reluctance his parents agreed that they would not lock the tent, but moved it into their own bedroom where William could sleep in it without the lock and be monitored by them until his bedroom was transformed into a 'safe area', including additional padding on the walls and making safe windowsills and windows, using a Disabled Facilities Grant.

See Chapter 11 for the other intervention that was put in place with the family and an activity for you to complete about William.

It is essential that social workers, their managers and other professionals are mindful of the requirement to understand the level of need and risk in a family from the child's perspective, and ensure that actions which will have maximum impact on the child's life are explored. No system can fully eliminate risk. Understanding risk involves judgment and balance. To manage risks, social workers and other professionals should make decisions with the best interests of the child in mind, informed by the evidence available and underpinned by knowledge of child development. Critical reflection through supervision should strengthen the analysis in each assessment (DfE 2015:24).

Taking it further

NSPCC – National Society for the Prevention of Cruelty to Children (2003) 'It Doesn't Happen to Disabled Children: Child Protection and Disabled Children'. *Report of the National Working Group on Child Protection and Disability.* London: NSPCC. Available online www.nspcc.org.uk/preventing-abuse/child-abuse-and-neglect/child-sexual-abuse/ (accessed 20 April 2016).

NCA CEOP – National Crime Agency and Child Exploitation and Online Protection Centre http://ceop.police.uk/About-Us/ (accessed). This website has a section specifically for social workers: http://ceop.police.uk/Knowledge-Sharing/charities/ (accessed 5 January 2016).

Erooga, M and Print B Assessing parental capacity when intrafamilial sexual abuse by an adult is a concern, in *The Child's World: Assessing Children in Need*, J Horwath (ed). London: Jessica Kingsley Publishers Ltd, pp 303–320, including 'Finkelhor (1984) model of sexual abuse', pp 314–315.

Link for fabricated illness and real life example:

Community Care Social workers' role in cases of fabricated illness www.communitycare.co.uk/2010/06/04/social-workers-role-in-cases-of-fabricated-illness/ (accessed 10 September 2015).

Further research and statistics about children with disabilities can be found on the Contact a Family website:

Contact a Family Research www.cafamily.org.uk/professionals/research/ (accessed 19 August 2015).

PREVENT

H M Government (2015) *Revised Prevent duty guidance for England and Wales: Guidance for specified authorities in England and Wales on the duty in the Counter-Terrorism and Security Act 2015 to have due regard to the need to prevent people from being drawn into terrorism.* Norwich: The Stationery Office. Available online www.gov.uk/government/uploads/system/uploads/attachment_data/file/445977/3799_Revised_Prevent_Duty_Guidance_England_Wales_V2-Interactive.pdf (accessed 15 December 2015).

Home Office and DfE guidance How Social Media is used to encourage Travel to Syria and Iraq: briefing note for schools www.emcsrv.com/prolog/PG/DfE/Schools_Guide-Social_Media_V16.pdf and www.preventforschools.org/?category_id=55 (accessed 15 December 2015).

Chapter 3 | Managing the emotional impact of disability

This chapter gives you a brief look at a subject that can be very difficult and emotive, both in your personal life and as a social worker. When you are dealing with loss and grief, particularly associated with death or dying, it can bring about emotions that will take you back to deep feelings that you may have experienced, or be experiencing, in your personal life. This chapter gives you some techniques to help you deal with difficult conversations and to understand the cycle of grief and loss that many children and families you work with will be experiencing. It also discusses advanced care planning. We take a brief look at emotional intelligence and resilience and why these are important to us as social workers. We explore why you need to look after your own emotional intelligence in order to safely manage complex subjects such as life-limiting conditions. We also briefly examine how our emotions play a part in our communication, which is particularly important when working with people with learning disabilities and their families.

Grief and loss

Loss is experienced differently by everyone and there are no rules or right or wrong about how to deal with it. Loss comes in many different shapes and does not only have to be the death of a loved one. Loss can be, for example, the loss of a relationship, a limb, a job, aspirations, your support network, empty nest syndrome, financial loss, the loss of one or more of your senses, loss of personal belongings from a fire or loss of your health. Obviously this list is not exhaustive, and we would all feel and act differently if we experienced these things in our lives.

It is important to remember when working with parents and other family members of children with disabilities that they may be experiencing grief and loss. This may be, for example, at the point of diagnosis when parents are told their child, whom they had lots of hopes and aspirations for, has a disability and will never be able to achieve the things that many of us take for granted, or when they are told their child's disability is degenerative or that an illness is terminal.

Activity: **Loss at diagnosis**

Think about the host of losses, feelings and emotions that would be experienced by parents, grandparents and siblings when a child in their family is diagnosed with a disability. Remember that some of these feelings may be uncomfortable to admit.

Recently diagnosed child

When a family has to face a diagnosis around their child's disability, you need to consider this holistically, and think about the ramifications for each individual within the family. There are the obvious 'losses' for the individual at the centre of the diagnosis. Depending upon the diagnosis and its complexities, the person given the diagnosis may not yet have an understanding of what it means for them, nor may they ever. If diagnosed as a baby or at a young age, it could be years before they do understand and consider their losses. For example, it may not be until the child goes to school that they begin to see their individual differences or that they are unable to do the same things as their peers.

Siblings

Siblings will deal with issues differently depending upon their position in the family. For example, the firstborn child does not have a disability and adapts well to the arrival of a new brother or sister, but then has to deal with the emotional impact of having a sibling with a disability; or perhaps they are a twin and the other twin has a disability; or a second sibling is born and there is already a child with a disability in the family. Siblings will need support and must be given careful consideration as to their own needs. You should also bear in mind that a sibling of a child with a disability may already, or in the future, be a young carer and as a result of this may experience 'loss' of part of their childhood due to their additional responsibilities. They may also experience loss because their parents are less able to meet their needs due to the demands of their sibling's disability, and because the needs of the child with the disability have to take priority, for example when planning activities and days out. There is the additional loss associated with not having a 'normal' sibling relationship, playing together and the natural sibling rivalry that you share, particularly if the disability is severe and profound with complex health needs. On the other hand, having a sibling with a disability might enhance your relationship with that special person and enrich your life. We consider siblings further in this chapter, and in Chapter 6.

There are support groups such as Spurgeons (www.spurgeons.org/). They support young carers and give them the opportunity to be a child again, taking time off from their caring role and responsibilities.

Grandparents

Grandparents are often an essential and vital support in the family but can be a forgotten generation and their own needs easily overlooked. They will experience loss in ways that they too find difficult to come to terms with. They have the worry for their child (ie a parent of the child with the disability) and the additional worry for their grandchild and may be overwhelmed by grief for both generations. They may also be left out when it comes to receiving information about their grandchild's condition and how best to manage it, or feel overwhelmed with too much information and an expectation that they will take a hands-on role in the care of the child. This could involve complex training regimes, which they may feel afraid to decline for fear of being ostracised and seen as uncaring. Some hospices hold Grandparent Days to give them support and allow them time to share their feelings and worries. Some younger grandparents may be the 'sandwich' generation, who have additional responsibilities supporting and caring for their own elderly parents as well as having a grandchild with a disability, and may feel torn when they have to choose who to help or try and stretch themselves to help everyone.

There are additional feelings that family members may have to face when there are genetic conditions and the associated blame that goes alongside this, 'I've passed this on to my child, it's my fault.'

When working with a family who have just received a diagnosis, you need to remember that each family member will be in a different place emotionally and managing things differently. They may not understand some of the feelings they are experiencing or why other family members are not feeling the same way as them. They may even think the other people in their family are not feeling any grief or have moved on.

Death of a child

Death is the biggest loss we experience in our lives, but even death is sometimes expected and seen as part of the natural cycle of life. It can be easier to cope with the death of someone who has had a long and full life and when death is expected. The loss of a child is not accepted in the same way, and nor should it be. A parent does not expect to have to mourn their own child.

When a parent has a child with a complex health need or disability it is a reality they may be dealing with now or have to face in the future. They may have been told that their child's condition is terminal but often a child's life expectancy can be difficult to determine; however, there are times when you will be working with a family whose child is close to death or who has recently died.

Cycle of change associated with grief and loss

One of the pioneers of research and models of support and counselling for dealing with trauma and grief and the grieving process was Elizabeth Kübler-Ross, who in 1969 published her book *On Death and Dying*. Kübler-Ross developed a five-stage model showing the critical journey travelled by those who have experienced trauma, including death. These five stages are transferable to different aspects of life, and individuals experience the stages at different degrees.

Let's have a look at Kübler-Ross' model. Leading up to the start of the five stages is the shock from the loss or incident.

The Five Stages

1. Denial – unable to accept what has happened.

2. Anger – this can show itself in many ways. Some people will become upset and cry a lot or become withdrawn, while others may show their anger by physical or aggressive outbursts.

3. Bargaining – this is when you face up to the trauma or loss you have experienced. You may make 'deals' with yourself to get through this time or begin to come to terms with the reality of the situation and its finality.

4. Depression – the realisation that things will never be the same again and you prepare for what is ahead. You move towards acceptance but are still upset and emotional. You may have feelings of hopelessness and an 'emptiness' in your life, and you may regret things that were not said. This is 'preparatory grieving'.

5. Acceptance – this stage will come at different times depending upon the type and extent of the loss. You will start to feel stronger and begin to emotionally detach yourself from the person you have lost (Kübler-Ross 1973).

When you are working with families who are dealing with trauma and loss, including death and dying, you must respect an individual's perspective and the way they are managing their situation. A child may die, and each person who knows that child, whether it be a parent, sibling, uncle, cousin, grandmother, teacher, friend or neighbour, will show their emotional responses in different ways, depending on their own life experiences.

Each person will spend different amounts of time at each stage, and as they accept the reality of their loss, they will be able to move forward and manage their day-to-day life. This is obviously a simplistic view of this roller coaster of emotions, and as you will know from your own life challenges and traumas, when you are actually in this cycle it is often difficult to accept it when people say to you that 'time heals'.

The Dual Process Model of grief and loss

Another model that will help you understand how people deal with grief and loss is the Dual Process Model (Stroebe and Schut 1999). It recognises that people experience the stages of grief differently, with some people being 'loss-orientated' while others are 'restoration-orientated'. Those who are loss-orientated tend to have feelings of grief, such as loneliness, sadness, emptiness, anger, confusion and depression, and may be dealing with anticipatory loss and fears of loss of their future. Those who are in the restoration-orientated mode are often looking at the here and now and dealing with day-to-day issues, but not looking to the future or planning ahead; they are trying to manage the situation but may be avoiding the grief. They will focus on new things or divert from grief by making new friends, continuing with hobbies etc, but after doing 'nice' or 'normal' things they feel guilty for having some happiness.

People often switch between the two models, sometimes consciously but also unconsciously, depending on what is happening in their life. Switching between the two models helps people cope and gives them permission to have the happy feelings that while in the grief process you feel guilty for having. It is important to remember that those are the moments that help keep people sane and able to carry on each day. Taking time off from the grief gives parents and carers the strength to keep going when caring for a child with a disability.

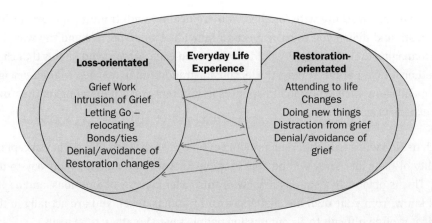

Stroebe, M and Schut, H (1999) The Dual Process Model of Coping with Bereavement: Rationale and Description, *Death Studies*, 23:3, 197–224, used with permission from Taylor & Francis. Available online http://dx.doi.org/10.1080/074811899201046 (accessed 30 May 2015).

Advanced care planning

A Child and Young Person's Advanced Care Plan (ACP) is designed to communicate the wishes and feelings of a child or young person who is deemed to be in palliative care or who has a life-limiting condition. The document identifies a plan, agreed by the child (depending upon their ability to contribute, development, age and stage) and their family setting out their feelings about actions that should be taken when the child's condition becomes life-threatening.

Everyone who has an important role to play in a child or young person's life can be involved with setting out the agreed plan that will be followed for that child should their condition deteriorate. As their social worker, you may have important information to contribute towards the plan and therefore may be involved both at the planning stage and at a review.

It is important to remember that the ACP can be used as a resuscitation plan and not just for the end of life, and also be used in different settings, ie for the child to take to school so that all the teaching staff involved with the child are aware of how to respond in particular circumstances.

There are many legalities associated with advanced care planning and considerations may be given, for example, to 'Do Not Attempt Cardiopulmonary Resuscitation (DNACPR)'. Decisions such as place of death will be considered by the family, and parents will sometimes choose to be with their child at a hospice when the time comes rather than their child being cared for at home. Hospice staff are highly trained in dealing with all issues related to end of life care, and there are special facilities, such as end of life suites, where families can stay with their child until after they have died.

The ACP for a child is different to that used for an adult; the two statutes underpinning the plans are the Mental Capacity Act 2005, which is the test used for capacity, and the Children Act 1989. The Children Act 1989 will give consideration to what is in the *'child's best interests'*. These two pieces of legislation need to be used in parallel. There are many issues to consider regarding decisions around capacity and whether a young person is deemed to be Gillick competent and/or meets the Fraser guidelines, ie is capable of making certain decisions. *'At 16 a young person can be presumed to have capacity to consent; a young person under 16 may have the capacity to consent, depending upon their ability to understand'* (General Medical Council 2010: 48). The Mental Capacity Act 2005, particularly for young people aged 16 and 17, is specific to individual decisions that the person is making; a young person may lack the capacity to make a major decision such as whether they want a DNACPR, but they may be able to make a decision about where they wish to be at the end of their life, ie at home or in a hospice etc.

Professionals involved in writing and overseeing ACPs will have received comprehensive training, and you would not be the lead professional but may have to contribute to the plan. Talking to children with palliative medical conditions is complex, and the discussions need to be managed sensitively. The child may be fearful about death and dying and find it easier to talk to you about this rather than their parents. Use language they can understand (Bennett 2012). Think about how you might react to what a child may ask or tell you about and consider your responses, but be honest with them: you will need to use your emotional intelligence. Many children with complex health needs and disabilities will not be able to express their wishes and feelings. It is essential that you can deal with the enormous emotional implications of working within this most sensitive area of social work and healthcare. You can help families enormously just by being a good, active listener and offering emotional support at this time, but do not get personally involved and if necessary redirect the family to organisations that can offer this support, such as Cruse Bereavement Care or Child Bereavement UK (www. crusebereavementcare.org.uk or www.childbereavement.org.uk).

The ACP will consider dignity, respect and compassion and should also consider an individual's social, ethnic, cultural, psychological, spiritual and religious beliefs. You must respect families' decisions and their values and ethics even if they differ from your own. You will perhaps not know the minutiae between different cultural groups and communities. For example, there are many differences with regard to the rituals and ceremonies different religions observe at the time of death and immediately afterwards. The Hindu community will hold a funeral very quickly, usually a cremation within 24 hours of the child's death (or as soon as possible after registering the death), and the Jewish community would also hold a burial within 24 hours of death, unless the death is on the Sabbath (Saturday) or another holy day (Bennett 2012). It may not be up to you to consider all the cultural issues, but you can discuss them with other professionals involved prior to talking to families if this is an identified task for you to do.

Upon completion of an ACP it is signed by parent(s) (or person holding parental responsibility) and a senior doctor/clinician who knows the child and has been part of the planning process. The plan must be shared with all professionals who are routinely involved with the child's care (ie, within all the different settings they attend). It should also be shared with anyone who may be contacted at the time of an emergency, ie local ambulance departments. This allows everyone to be aware of the wishes and feelings of the child and family when the time comes to put the plan into action. ACPs are regularly reviewed to ensure that everyone is still in agreement with all aspects of them; the timing of such reviews would depend on the needs of the individual child but should be regular enough to ensure that the plan remains current.

Managing difficult conversations when dealing with grief and loss

As discussed earlier you will need to remember that people will be at different stages of the grieving process, and this can make communication difficult. One parent may be loss-orientated and another somewhere within the restoration-orientated stage, resulting in a loss of understanding between them. This will bring its own tension and may create conflict that has not previously been experienced within the family unit or relationship. In conjunction with this there may be siblings who are experiencing their own difficulties and may not understand why their mother and father are at loggerheads or why everyone is sad – they may even be blaming themselves for the loss of their sibling. The issues are very complex.

Activity: **Things to consider**

You have just been allocated a new case, and you find that the family have just been given a diagnosis or have to come to terms with the realities of making an Advanced Care Plan for their child. It is your job to undertake an assessment of need to ascertain the support that is required. Think about what you may have to consider when undertaking your assessment visit. Here are a few things to start you off:

» *Who has not accepted the reality of the situation?*

» *Who is still trying to process their feelings and responses to the new situation they find themselves in?*

» *Who is adjusting to the reality? And how are they demonstrating this?*

» *Are the ways the parents/carers are having to relate to their child different to what they had expected?*

» *Is the parent/carer able to build relationships with professionals?*

» *Are they focusing on the here and now and not the future? Are they able to 'enjoy the moment'? Is this perhaps stopping them from accepting the future?*

You will have to manage and facilitate difficult conversations with families throughout your career as a social worker, but particularly when dealing with these types of situations. Families want to know that you understand their grief and what they are going through, even if you don't and hopefully will never have to experience the pain of losing a child or having a child being diagnosed with a disability. You should be empathic and understanding but not be too sympathetic and emotional yourself. They will be coming to terms with difficult decisions they have to make or that have already been made. They might be adjusting to not hearing their child's voice again or being able to have conversations with their child due to their disability. Parents may not want to talk to you and have to explain their situation, or they may have had to tell their story numerous times already, but it is important that you are able to coax out the information you need. Often families say they are managing their situation and they don't want to cause a fuss; some are very resilient at these times and will use their own support networks, which is always preferable.

Remember:

» Clarify exactly what is being said and be clear about what you are being told. You may often have to interrupt the parent to ask for more detail.

» Paraphrase to ensure that you show your understanding.

» Make sure you are emotionally strong enough to manage these conversations, and if you find yourself going to a place in your mind that is 'dark' and too painful due to your own experiences, try to manage this carefully and when appropriate perhaps steer the conversation to another area.

» It may be useful to have a packet of tissues nearby to give to the parent/carer but be careful not to give the message that you are giving them the tissue to stop them crying. Crying is an outlet for the storyteller and a natural part of the grieving process. They may need to cry or it may be the first time that the person has opened up and been able to cry. You should let them know that this is OK, and they can cry. It is never a sign of being weak.

» Ensure you have a debrief with your manager afterwards.

If anger is manifesting itself, try to manage this sensitively and de-escalate it via acknowledgement; however, if this anger is becoming out of control you need to risk assess the situation and ensure that you and others are safe. You may need to end the conversation. If the anger is felt to be 'safe' and not escalating, it needs to come out and be accepted that this is an understandable behaviour linked to grief. This may be the only way the person knows how to express their feelings.

Silence can be very difficult or uncomfortable to deal with, but it can be productive to a person taking time to process the information they have been given or make sense of what is going on in their world. Try not to be uncomfortable with the silence and, when appropriate, try to read their body language to gently re-engage the person in dialogue. Being silent doesn't mean that they have disengaged and if they are looking down or away from you or out of the window you may just need to give them more time; however, if they do look towards you they may be looking to you to break the silence and restart the conversation. When you are dealing with silences, be aware of your own body language and facial expressions: remain engaged and approachable, don't be poker-faced or dismissive.

Below we list some factors that can help make difficult conversations and communication more successful:

» Remember it's a two-way process

» Acceptance and clarity of issues and the situation

» Being a good facilitator

» The person sees you are listening and interested

» Using simple, easy language

» Using active listening skills and paraphrasing and summarising

» Open body language – being aware of non-verbal signs and language

» Time management – enough time to maximise potential but not overkill

» Good endings – planning and managing this

» Awareness of self

» Being focused

» Open and closed questioning

» Calm environment

» Comfortable with silences and different emotions being shown

Getting the most out of your conversations

When you are talking to parents and carers, don't make them feel that they have to talk to you for hours on end – you need to recognise when they have had enough. But, while you *are* able to talk to them and they are open to the discussion, it is key to ensure that you are using useful phrases and questioning techniques to help them give you the information you want. Use phrases like:

Tell me more about…

What do you mean by…

That's an interesting point (question/comment), what makes you ask/say that?

What is your understanding about…

When you say that, how do you feel…

What are your reasons for saying that?

What would (eg husband, wife, other child, grandparent) say about… (Use the phrase for each important member of the family/network as necessary).

How did you manage this…

How did you feel at that time… (again asking each person involved)

Consider what makes conversations challenging. What is difficult for you may not be difficult for someone else. It is always best practice to plan your visits and think about what you need to cover and achieve. If you are co-working with another member of your team you may know how that person works, and if you work well together this process may not be difficult. If you are working with someone you don't know, it is a good idea to get together beforehand and look at how you are going to collaborate during the visit. Discuss your own knowledge and experience of the family and if there are likely to be any areas of conflict. This is important if you are going to see a family who are in a heightened state of anxiety, particularly if you or another worker has had a previous negative experience with them.

Conversations are usually challenging when you are giving bad news. Be careful about anticipating conversations too much; they may start well but go in unexpected directions and then conclude unsatisfactorily. Remember, you may experience a range of reactions and these may not always be what you expected. Don't use sarcasm.

Take a few moments to consider the following:

» The range of reactions you might witness and how you would respond.

» Which situations you find the most difficult to deal with.

Ask yourself:

» Am I the right person to have this particular conversation?

» Should I be having the conversation on my own, or do I need someone else in the room?

Acknowledge the difficulties of the conversation.

Be clear about expectations.

Talking to siblings

Siblings are often plunged into the cruel reality of their family situation very quickly. Regardless of their age they may feel out of control, frightened and out of their depth. They may feel angry or guilty and blame themselves, or feel that they have to take control and be strong or just stay quiet and not say anything. They will feel exactly the same as everyone else but may not understand why they have these feelings or how they manifest themselves in different ways, such as having 'tummy aches'. They may be hearing lots of medical language and words they do not understand.

Children are often aware that things are 'going on' around them, and that when they walk into a room it goes quiet or they are sent to their bedroom while adults talk. They know that information is being withheld and this again may make them feel alone, and more frightened. Depending upon their age and understanding they may feel that their parents are not being honest with them and are holding things back. This could result in the sibling making things up and fantasising about what may have happened: this could be more frightening than the truth.

A child's understanding of and reaction to a situation will be affected by many things, including their age and stage of development, what they have been told by the adults around them, what they have overheard from other people (perhaps when their parents think they are out of earshot) and the impact of what may have happened in the child's daily life and the forced changes to their routine. A child might need help to express their feelings or worries. Someone needs to be communicating with them and help them understand what is going on. If their sibling has died or has to spend periods of time out of the family home – perhaps in hospital or in a hospice – they will need to know where their sibling is, what is happening and why. Children may have a better understanding than you think. They often ask questions and will usually cope with the answers. If you are faced with this, it is important to agree with their parents about what the child is to be told.

If a sibling asks, 'Is my brother going to die?', you might reply 'What makes you say that?' to gauge their understanding of the situation before answering. Don't overload the child with too much information at once: break it down into manageable chunks and be guided by the child. They may accept what you tell them and not ask you anything further. If they ask something that you don't know the answer to, it is OK to say this and explain that sometimes grown-ups don't always know the answer and that they too struggle to understand what is happening. If a child asks you something as the social worker and you are not sure what response to give, you can say 'Let's see what mum and dad think about that...' as it is essential to liaise with them and work together, and that the sibling's questions are not ignored. Again, however, this may be very difficult if the parents are at different places in their own acceptance of the situation or the grief cycle.

A starting point to help a child understand may be doing an 'illustration'. The exact nature of this illustration will vary based on the child's age, stage and any disability; it may need to be very simple. You could develop the illustration to explain the situation to the child who has been given the diagnosis or their sibling(s) or both. There are different ways of delivering this information and you need to discuss and agree with parents what information you are sharing. (Illustrations are explored further in Chapter 4.)

The illustration shown gives a snapshot to Charlie's sibling about what has happened and what it is likely to happen in the near future while Charlie is in hospital and when he comes home. This gives an age-appropriate 'snapshot' to Charlie's sibling without overloading him/her with too much complex information. Another illustration could be completed as things change.

Illustration: Charlie's story, so far

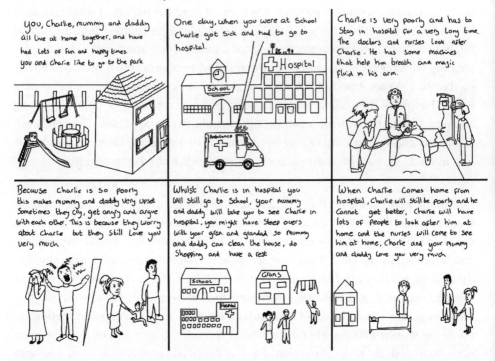

You, Charlie, mummy and daddy all live at home together, and have had lots of fun and happy times. You and Charlie like to go to the park.

One day, when you were at School Charlie got sick and had to go to hospital.

Charlie is very poorly and has to stay in hospital for a very long time. The doctors and nurses look after Charlie. He has some machines that help him breath and magic fluid in his arm.

Because Charlie is so poorly this makes mummy and daddy very upset. Sometimes they cry, get angry and argue with each other. This is because they worry about Charlie but they still love you very much.

Whilst Charlie is in hospital you will still go to School, your mummy and daddy will take you to see Charlie in hospital, you might have sleep overs with your gran and grandad so mummy and daddy can clean the house, do shopping and have a rest.

When Charlie comes home from hospital, Charlie will still be poorly and he cannot get better, Charlie will have lots of people to look after him at home and the nurses will come to see him at home, Charlie and your mummy and daddy love you very much.

Having something on paper (or more likely perhaps it can be completed on an electronic device such as the child's tablet) allows the child to save the illustration and look at it later. They can initiate conversations by bringing the illustration to you when they feel like talking about the situation, or read it in private.

You may also want to make a 'worry box' for the child for them to empty all their worries into to help get them out of their head. There are many variations of the worry box you can explore and individualise for each child.

You can help families by talking to them about 'memory boxes' that they can put together to keep their memories of the special times they had with the child who is dying or who may have already passed away. If the family are able to discuss the issues early on, they can start to think about which key times they want to capture. It is much easier in the digital age to take photos but sometimes families may want to keep more tangible mementos, including collecting keepsakes, hand and foot prints of their child and other things that will bring fond memories. Later you could discuss other ways of remembering the deceased, such as planting a special tree.

Many of the conversations will not be easy. You need to be honest, but balancing hope with realism is difficult, especially as children do need to feel that they will be 'alright'.

After difficult conversations, ensure you take any issues to your own supervisor and debrief. Make sure you engage in 'reflective practice exercises', exploring which aspects of the conversation you think went well, what might you have done more of, and what could you have done differently? This isn't so you beat yourself up about anything that didn't go quite to plan, but to firstly, and importantly, allow you to build your own resilience and talk through your feelings to ensure you are not left with the family's stress; this is known as 'vicarious trauma'. Secondly, it is to help you learn and talk through any difficulties you experienced, and to understand why some parts of the conversation may have been more difficult than others. As already discussed, this could be due to your own experiences being brought to the forefront.

Emotional intelligence

Emotional intelligence (EQ) is different to an intelligence quotient or IQ. There are several models of emotional intelligence that have been developed since the 1920s, but Daniel Goleman's 1995 book, *Emotional Intelligence: Why it can matter more than IQ*, is generally regarded as the flagship text on the subject.

Goleman identified five areas of emotional intelligence:

»   motivation

»   empathy

»   self-awareness

»   self-regulation

»   social skills.

We believe all these elements are essential for social workers, particularly when working in this specialist field.

»   Motivation – your drive to persist in order to achieve your goal

»   Empathy – understanding and giving consideration to other people's emotions and feelings

»   Self-awareness – knowing and understanding your moods and emotions and their effects on others

»   Self-regulation – controlling and regulating emotions, including negative and disruptive emotions

»   Social skills – managing relationships and networking with others to achieve desired outcomes

Goleman believed that EQ is a learnt behaviour and can be developed. We hope that this chapter provides you with the key skills to help you to develop your own EQ, which you can add to your toolkit of knowledge and skills to draw upon in difficult situations.

Understanding your emotions

Emotional intelligence is a key to understanding and communicating with people, particularly children with learning difficulties and those who are non-verbal. Our emotions affect how we communicate even if we don't always realise it. We communicate by the way we stand or sit, through our facial expressions and gestures or by how we respond to someone. It is important to recognise what someone is saying with their body language, which allows us to communicate in a way that is 'honest' in that it is natural; often the person you are communicating with will not be consciously aware of the messages they are sending out. Using our EQ allows us to recognise these traits (Hasson 2012).

Once you have considered these things it is important to think about your own emotions and how you are responding to the other person. Just for a moment, think about how we often 'mirror' others' body language when we are talking to them. If they fold their arms or cross their legs, we will often, without realising, do the same. We all have emotional responses that are both positive and negative and which can change very quickly. You need to understand your own emotions and be aware of them. If you have just received some really good news for example, it would not be appropriate to go singing and dancing into a meeting about advanced care planning with a family who are about to discuss their child's end of life care. Neither do you have to be sad and scared to smile or acknowledge that you have had some good news, but this has to be appropriate and sensitive. You need to recognise how your own emotions affect others around you. If you are preoccupied, for example about your good news, and your emotions are running high you will not be able to concentrate on the task at hand and process what is being said properly: others may therefore think you are insensitive and uncaring.

Knowing what type of person you are will help you. Being honest about your assessment of yourself will also help you understand your and other people's emotions. Are you a glass half empty or half full type of person; a radiator who 'radiates' positive energy; or a 'drain' who drains away people's positive energy by being moody or always complaining about something? We are influenced by those around us and their mood. Have you noticed how the atmosphere in a room can change just by one person entering or leaving it? By using your EQ, it will help you become more aware of who influences you and importantly how this may change your own behaviour. Consider how other people can affect your mood and how you can in turn use positive emotions and responses to influence others. You cannot make everything better by trying to be happy all the time but by understanding and using your EQ you will help get more from others.

Consider the following points:

- » Acknowledge that you may need to change and why (admit if you are the drain, learn to understand why and ask yourself – do I need to change?)
- » Think about your body language and read the other person's
- » Give appropriate eye contact – don't stare
- » The tone of your voice and the language you use
- » Try and find something positive in any given situation
- » Ask what worked well in the past
- » Engage in active listening (nod, acknowledge, reflect and paraphrase)
- » Empathise with people
- » Put effort into conversations and show interest
- » Acknowledge someone's situation/grief/happiness/feelings
- » Stay motivated
- » Understand how the situation is affecting you, and your responses to others
- » Become more aware of and listen to your intuition.

Now you have some understanding of the basics of emotional intelligence, you can link this to your practice. We believe this is essential when you are working with children and adults who have complex health needs and learning difficulties, and their families, because you are often dealing with emotive situations.

Being emotionally intelligent and recognising your emotions will make you more resilient.

Scenario: A roller coaster day at work

One day I was asked to go to a hospice to support a family in the end of life suite. I came face-to-face with a child who had died some days ago, with their parents lying beside them, not having left the room, cuddling and kissing their child while

> *sobbing constantly and not wanting to let go of their child. I was experiencing and witnessing the agonising pain of the parents' grief and loss. I had to draw upon the skills needed to balance professionalism, strength and empathy: my role was to be there with them and be their emotional support. On returning to the office still carrying these difficult images and emotions, I received a call from a distressed mother who was crying and upset because her son with Asperger's wouldn't get out of bed and go to school. This conversation lasted 55 minutes, with the mother at breaking point and becoming increasingly angry with me; much of her distress was targeted at previous social workers and the team manager, who in the mother's opinion had 'let her down' and caused her distress. These repeated outbursts about her experience of social care were a 'cycle' the mother would often revert to when distressed.*

Although the first point of this scenario is an extreme example and one that the author has only had to deal with once in their social care career, it evidences the unexpected nature of social work when dealing with children with complex health issues and limited life conditions. Although the parents' experiences in the scenario cannot be compared, each of the parent's pains and stresses are important to them, and while the grief and loss places a heavy load on you, you still need to respond to the parents who appear to have the more trivial problem.

Emotional intelligence and resilience when balanced well will enable you to switch and adapt your responses to meet the needs of individual situations. There is no book or plan to tell you how to do this: you need to trust in your intuition and have the awareness of where you are at in terms of EQ. This is the foundation that helps to build the resilience you will need in this role.

Resilience

Resilience is another word for how we deal with stress and the demands placed upon us in our lives – having the ability to 'bounce back'. There are many different pressures on us, for example, being a parent, a carer for a relative, having a job and running a home to name a few. Being able to positively manage these pressures and stressors is being resilient. This does not mean that we have to be Superman or Superwoman, and we cannot always manage every situation in a positive way. We may for example have difficulties in our home life at some time or another and have to manage situations that make our stress levels rise quickly, but at the same time we are able to manage stressors at work much more easily, or vice versa. It is said that much of how we deal with stress and our ability to cope is linked with our genetics and innate responses, either being a positive person who looks on the bright side and is very optimistic, or someone who is more sensitive to stress. Our resilience, however, is also linked with our experiences, particularly our early attachments and relationships, but we also develop resilience as we travel along life's pathways and learn from its knocks and triumphs. Those people with good support networks and who have developed close friendships are more resilient, and having a positive self-image coupled with higher self-esteem helps promote resilience both in our own lives and that of others, as you can help others manage their emotions and hopefully bring about positive changes (Howe 2008).

Children who are nurtured and have secure attachments usually deal more success-fully with stressful situations than those in neglectful situations/families. Stress can run high in families where there are children with disabilities for all of the reasons mentioned above; however, even during the very difficult times most children will have a bank of happy, secure and loving experiences that will help pull them through the difficult days.

Parents can help promote resilience in their children's lives (and their own) by mod-elling resilient behaviour, such as providing unconditional positive regard, love, trust and emotional support, and creating structure and routines in the child's day-to-day life, with rules that make them feel safe. Parents should encourage their child to become more independent and autonomous, exposing them to appropriate risk and giving them responsibility to build their confidence. It is important to allow children to build their self-esteem and be proud of their own achievements. Parents need to communicate with their children and encourage them to talk about their feelings and listen to them. This allows children to understand their own behaviour and emotions, and dependent on their age and understanding it will promote their comprehension of what is going on around them. It is good for children to know that although at times they will experience high stress levels, with love and security around them they will overcome the difficult times. Being exposed to *some* stress actually promotes resili-ence and well-being, and personal growth is enhanced.

Being aware of your own stress levels and how your job as a social worker can affect your emotions is important. You need to consider how you release your tension and stress in order to have a healthy mind and body. See Adams and Sheard (below) for further information about stress, work-life balance and emotional intelligence.

Taking it further

Adams, J and Sheard, A (2013) *Positive Social Work: The Essential Toolkit for NQSWs*, St Albans: Critical Publishing (Chapter 5 and Chapter 7). Also see page 47 where you can 'test' your own emotional intelligence.

Bennett, H (August 2012) *A Guide to End of Life Care of Children and Young People Before Death, at the Time of Death and After Death.* Bristol: Together for Short Lives. www.togetherforshortlives.org.uk.

Fraser et al (2011) *Life-Limiting Conditions in Children in the UK*, Division of Epidemiology, University of Leeds

Goleman, D (1996) *Emotional Intelligence: Why it can matter more than IQ*, London: Bloomsbury

Howe, D (2008) *The Emotionally Intelligent Social Worker*, Hampshire: Palgrave Macmillan

The Childhood Bereavement Network (CBN) for those working with bereaved children, young people and their families across the UK: www.childhoodbereavementnetwork.org.uk

A guide to developing good practice in childhood bereavement services (The Childhood Bereavement Network, 2006)

Chapter 4 | The child's voice: Exploring their world using good communication

This chapter explores communication, which is an essential part of working with children with disabilities. It is key to building your relationship and exploring the child's world and importantly, making sure the child's voice is heard by others. This chapter can only give you a tiny peek into the different methods and strategies for communication but we hope it fills you with inspiration and motivation to find out more. We briefly explore sensory disabilities and useful strategies for engaging with hearing and visually impaired children and young people. Different tools are explored such as Makaton and objects of reference, and we look at how you can use illustrations and other methods to communicate with children and give them a voice.

Think about when you are working with children with disabilities and how many of them will have difficulty communicating. Some may have a large vocabulary but others may not have any verbal communication at all, instead using sounds, cries (or babble), body language or hand and facial gestures that only people who know them well can understand, or at least pick out some of what they are trying to say. Some children may use signs or symbols and have a small selection of words they are familiar with and use with a trusted adult, such as 'hello', 'goodbye', 'yes', 'no', 'please' and 'thank you' while others may use assistive technology/electronic devices and drawings and illustrations – however they do it, remember they are still communicating.

Communication is a two-way process and a core social work skill regardless of which area you work in. Munro stated that:

Social workers sometimes feel inadequately trained to communicate with children. They may work with children of very varied ages, ethnicities, communication abilities and needs who require an equally varied range of skills in the social worker. Play and drawings may be more appropriate for some than anything resembling an interview... Training in communicating with children and young people can solve part of the problem. There are also a variety of tools that can be used to help children communicate their views. (Munro 2011:para 6.20 and 6.21:89)

Failing to understand communication is strongly linked with behavioural problems and challenging behaviour, and many children and young people with learning difficulties have problems with their communication. The more severe the difficulties, the more likely their communication is affected, thus the more likely difficult behaviour will escalate. This may be from being given too much information, the information not being delivered in the right way, or not being understood.

When planning any communication with children with disabilities it is important to consider:

- What is the 'expected' age and stage of development for a non-disabled child of the same age?
- What evidence do I have that the child has or has not reached that stage?
- What age and stage does the child actually mirror within their development?

You need to remember, however, that with many children with disabilities it is more complex than ages and stages: you have to consider the child's diagnosis too and how that affects their cognitive and physical development and barriers for learning etc. With some children it is very difficult on first meeting them to know how their disability affects their development. For example, a child may physically be functioning at an age-appropriate level, being able to walk, run or ride a bicycle, but cognitively they may not be at an equivalent stage. They may appear to understand what they are being asked or told but remember they may not have the ability to process the information and actually understand the different concepts, or their recall memory may be impaired. Just because they are capable of verbal communication it doesn't mean that the information they provide is reliable, and their responses may be out of context.

We are not going to discuss theories about learning and development here, but if you want to refresh your learning here are a few theorists you could explore: Bruner, Bowlby, Chomsky, Freud, Kohlberg, Piaget and Vygotsky. For a quick and simplistic overview, see Tim Gully in our 'Taking it further' section.

Why communicate, and how?

Communication is necessary for a child to be socially included and to become involved and participate actively in the things we ordinarily take for granted. The wider issues around social exclusion are often predominant features in the lives of children with disabilities and their families, who experience multiple exclusions, namely: socio-economic structural inequalities such as poverty and lack of access to the labour market; inappropriate housing; and a lack of co-ordinated and integrated services. They also face attitudinal barriers, direct and indirect discrimination and exclusion from services and lack of appropriate resources (Clarke 2006, Beresford and Rhodes 2008, Rix et al 2005 and Petrie et al 2007, cited in Mitchell et al 2009). These issues emphasise why it is so important that we work hard to ensure that we are able to hear, listen to and importantly, act on the child's voice, either by supporting them to do it, or by advocacy. Children with disabilities already face barriers and are disempowered by society and adults whether intentionally or not, and those children and young people who are non-verbal are even more likely to face an increased level of social exclusion and discrimination and be prevented from making decisions in their own lives.

It is important that you do your bit to ensure that you are actively communicating, breaking down barriers to communication and establishing the child's voice.

In order to communicate with a child with a disability (or any child), you need to think about the information you want to gain from the child. Ask yourself:

» What exactly is it that I want to know? (your objective)

» Why do I need this information? (for what purpose)

» What is the best way to gather this information? (what method will I use)

» What will I do with that information once I have it? (actions)

Also consider consent – is the child able to consent to sharing information with me? If not, who can do this on the child's behalf? Also ask, have I been open and honest with them about the questions above to inform their decision-making process?

Once that is clear, you should then consider how you intend to respond to the child, bearing in mind their disability and any complex needs, including health issues, that are associated with this. You should think about your own body language, facial expressions and how you make the child feel in your presence. Think about your language, tone of voice, and if necessary any symbols you wish to use. Do you have the correct symbols/signs for the situation? Will the child understand the signs you want to use? What other tools might you use? Dolls? Cars? Wii? iPad? You also need to consider how you are using your emotional intelligence, as discussed in Chapter 3.

Getting started

When starting a session with a child with disabilities, relax and remember this is a child first and foremost. Think about what you would do in the same circumstances but with a child who does not have a disability, then consider how their disability affects the child's communication. Don't be afraid of the child – this may sound silly but you would be surprised how often when you say a child has a disability, social workers suddenly forget all the skills they have for communicating with children and report the child has 'no communication'.

Remember, they don't have to be speaking, you have to 'read' them: their body language, gestures, hand signals, crying, vocalising or the blink of an eye. The slightest things should be taken into consideration and the child always praised for their efforts – it can be hard work for many young people. For example, a child using an eye gazer will need strength, patience and time to communicate with you. You must ensure that the child feels comfortable and is not rushed, otherwise they will become frustrated and upset and not engage with you. Also, let the child finish what they are trying to tell you – don't finish off their sentences for them because you are in a hurry or impatient. If you haven't got time then think carefully before starting any piece of work with a child because it would be very upsetting and hurtful if they were trying their very best to communicate with you and you said 'Sorry, I've got to go.' That would send the message that their voice was not worth hearing and they were not being listened to.

It is also important to have your 'safeguarding head' on too. Think about how the child is communicating with you:

- Are they presenting differently to usual? If so, how long have they been like this? Are they noticeably withdrawn when they are usually happy?
- What else might be contributing to this?
- How long has this been going on?
- Are they 'just not themselves', perhaps not giving you eye contact as they normally do or not responding to you in the usual way? Perhaps they are more apprehensive than usual.
- Are you instinctively feeling that something is not quite right?
- Are there any physical changes?

Talk to familiar adults about the child's presentation and reasons why things might have changed. We are not suggesting such changes necessarily mean there are any safeguarding concerns. The child may just be under the weather, having a difficult day or not have slept the previous night. Do consider that the child may be in physical pain but is unable to communicate this to you. Always think about what the child may be trying to communicate, and don't forget about safeguarding issues as a possible explanation – don't panic or raise unnecessary worry but talk to your manager if you are worried about any child protection concerns (see Chapter 2).

Here are a few things to think about that may help you to develop your skills:

» Explore the environment you wish to use for communicating with the child/ young person – is the lighting right? Is it quiet or noisy?

» Develop symbolic play and use your tools purposefully – for example, do you know how to use their chosen method of communication and understand it, ie Picture Exchange Communication System etc.

» Think about 'cause and effect' and how you are engaging with the child – are they able to pick up on your cues as well as you are picking up on theirs? What is happening when you are communicating with the child? Are you making progress?

» Are you actually listening to the child? Keep asking yourself this question. We don't mean just their voice (if the child is verbal). Watch how they are presenting – are they shuffling in their seat? If so, are they uncomfortable? Do they need attention to personal care? Are they unwell? Are they bored? Are they doing this because they are happy?

» What are your play skills like? Are you able to motivate the child and keep them interested to enable you to find out the information you require?

» Repeat instructions – small chunks depending upon their comprehension and understanding.

» You may need distraction techniques – think about how you will keep the child on task and keep them focused.

» Don't try and lead them – follow them first and gain their confidence.

» Be natural – don't try and be someone you are not. The child has to trust you and they will pick up on anything that they think is false.

» Keep giving praise and build their confidence – this helps build motivation. Smile – give good eye contact and face the child. Be gentle in your approach.

» If the child is autistic they may not understand certain phrases or will take things literally, for example something you are doing is funny – if you respond, 'I'm laughing my head off', they may think your head is actually going to come off!

» If you have to elicit some information from the child, think about their con-centration level – don't jump in too quickly with the questioning, but don't miss the opportunity either. Listen carefully to what you are being told and acknowledge it, but don't speak for them – don't put words into their mouth.

Research (Munro 2011) suggests we should see the child alone; this is not always possible when working with children with disabilities, but should be your aim when appropriate. You might need to have another person with you who is (a) familiar with the child's method of communication and who understands their gestures and man-nerisms and (b) trusted by the child. If this is a child protection case you need to think about who the most appropriate person is: it may not always be a parent if they are alleged perpetrators, so perhaps ask a teacher or one-to-one worker.

Methods of communication when working with children with disabilities

In Munro's final report in 2011, she discussed how adult voices were still being heard more than children's, and how children's voices were being missed in assessments and decisions that affected their lives. Therefore, before we go on to look at different methods to assist your communication with children with disabilities, think about how you might elicit information from James.

Activity: **Getting the most from James**

James is eight years old and has moderate learning disabilities. He attends a special school. He has a hearing impairment in one ear, epilepsy and selective mutism (this means that James has an anxiety disorder that prevents him from speaking in certain social situations such as school, but he is able to and does speak freely to close family and friends when nobody else is listening). You are undertaking an assessment of need and as part of this you are thinking about what types of short break James might like to take part in.

Draw up a plan showing how you might engage James in his assessment and what information you need from him. Think about things such as: what issues do you need to consider and what tools will you use? Which of your communication skills would you need to use most? Think about your own approach towards James and how you will need to conduct/present yourself. How many sessions might you need? Do you need help from anyone else?

To get a child or young person to engage with you and to help communication and break down the barriers there are different methods, including:

Play

Books and toys: there are a host of books available, some being more interactive than others. Find out what things the child is interested in and grab their attention by opening up communication through engaging them with pop-up or musical books. A visually impaired child may enjoy listening to audiobooks and the pop-up books that accompany them so they can touch and feel different textures etc. CDs can also be therapeutic too. Touch and feel toys are effective for children with sensory needs, including mirrors, coloured bubble tubes, kaleidoscopes and toys that they can squash or that squeak etc. Finger puppets and soft toys and dolls can also be enjoyed.

Once again remember that a child may not be functioning at their chronological age and therefore you may need use resources you would normally choose for younger children.

Games: There are a host of games you can use, from traditional games such as snakes and ladders, Frustration or card games, to computer games on eg Wii or PlayStation devices that can be fully interactional and cater for children with physical disabilities too.

Messy play is also enjoyed by children of all ages: sand pits, water play, painting and play dough. Children with autism often enjoy this more sensory play.

For those children who find it hard to concentrate, thus making communication more difficult, you may need to use distraction techniques and have different things in your 'tool box'. Some children may only be able to concentrate for a few short minutes before moving on to something else, so you only have limited opportunities to engage with them. Others prefer to play on their own or do not engage in play at all.

We don't expect you all to be 'play therapists', but remember that play offers many benefits for communicating with children and it can be great fun, too. We advise you to practise and practise – it's a great part of social work that we don't get to do as much as we should. Play allows you to have access to the child's world, even if only a sneaky peek. Play is a child's natural medium for expressing themselves and to experiment with the different ways they can learn. Play will help a child feel safe and secure and open up their communication channels and express themselves, letting their barriers down and thus showing their feelings and fears while helping stimulate their physical, emotional and social well-being. When playing with children, it is important to think about the setting and how you start the play. Get on the child's level – don't expect them to feel comfortable on a large chair that makes them look even smaller, the same way you would feel uncomfortable trying to sit in a child-sized chair. Perhaps sit on the floor with them, which will allow them to express themselves much better and is more child centred, putting you both on the same level. You must not be afraid to express yourself, throw away your inhibitions or let yourself look silly – honestly, it works. You also need to be patient. You need to build up trust with the child and:

- » Take things at the child's pace
- » Use child-friendly language
- » Use the child's preferred communication methods
- » Always be child focused and keep the child at the centre of everything

- » Respect the child

- » Chill out and be relaxed – don't try and be the boss

- » Have a selection of toys that you can use to interact with the child

- » Let the child lead you – they are the experts at playing, not you

Illustrations

Illustrations have been used to communicate with children (and adults) for many years. Story papers known in Britain as 'boys' weeklies' were very popular before the Second World War, with one well-known publication, *The Boy's Own Paper*, running from 1879 to 1967. There have been long-running publications such as *The Beano*, which was first published in 1937 and is still going today, and *The Dandy*, first published in 1938 (until 2012), which tell stories of mischievous acts and frolics to children of all ages. The point here is that this type of 'illustration' can be utilised within your work as a great way to engage with and tell a story to children. This idea has been developed in different aspects of social work with storyboards and 'Social Stories™', created by Carol Gray in 1991 in order to help teach social skills to children with autism, and the Signs of Safety model, which uses word and picture storyboards (Turnell and Essex 2006; Turnell and Edwards 2014) to create a narrative of events, primarily concerning child protection, for issues that adults find difficult to explain or discuss with children. There are other simplistic tools for helping children and adults with communication or learning difficulties, such as the Picture Exchange Communication System (PECS) and Makaton, which uses symbols. We are going to explore some of these later, but also see Chapter 3 for another example of using an illustration.

When putting an illustration together, think about why you need to tell the child this information, their age and understanding, their disability/impairment, what you want to tell the child, who is involved in the story and how you are going to break down the information into easy chunks. Are you going to involve the child in making the illustration, doing it together from the beginning, or are you going to do the illustration and present the story to the child afterwards? Do you need anyone else to help you to share this information and if so who will do what? Also, how will the child respond to the information? Remember, if the information is sensitive and it involves parents and/or other family members we advise you check with the parent/carer first to make sure they know what you are telling the child; the child may want to talk to them about it later and they may have to deal with any consequences or behaviour outbursts (if it is bad news) from the child.

Peter has atonic (drop) seizures and has to wear a helmet – his mother is explaining this to him.

Illustration: Wearing your helmet

Peter you Sometimes Fall because your body goes Floppy.

you call this 'having Wobbles.'

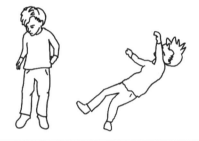

When you fall you might hurt yourself and bang your head.

This is dangerous when you hit your head 'having wobbles.'

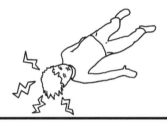

This means you have To wear your helmet when you go out So you don't hurt your head if you bang it.

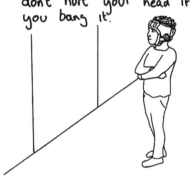

This is like when you and your friends ride your bicycles and you have a helmet to protect you.

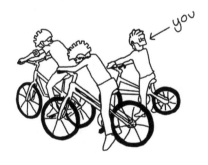

OK, now you can have a go at making an illustration for the following scenario. Remember not to use too many boxes – you don't want it too long or over-complicated.

Activity: **Going to short breaks**

Stuart is eight years old. He has some learning disabilities and it has just been identified that Stuart has some hearing impairment. Teachers are starting to introduce Stuart to some basic sign language. He has poor memory function and therefore can easily forget what he has been told and get confused about what is happening. He is showing some traits of autism and is currently undergoing assessment by CAMHS. His behaviour can be aggressive and he finds change difficult to deal with. You have completed a Social Care Assessment which identified that Stuart would benefit from short breaks at a local respite unit called 'Happy Stays'. The panel agreed to 12 overnight stays per year, therefore Stuart will go for one night each month. This will give Stuart the opportunity to have fun, a sleepover and meet new friends, while his parents (who are exhausted having to look after Stuart), get a well-earned rest. Stuart is due to go for his first introductory visit in two weeks' time and then have his first overnight the week after. His parents have asked that you tell Stuart this information as he likes you and looks forward to your visits. You are due to see him tomorrow.

Think about the points above and then put an illustration together to share with Stuart tomorrow.

Picture Exchange Communication System (PECS)

See more about PECS in Chapter 5, where we discuss methods and approaches for developing communication and learning for children with autism.

Objects of reference

Some children may have developed their own communication systems based on familiar objects that make them feel secure. They may have attached their own meaning to the object. For example, a child may have a 'snuggle' blanket that they get when they want to have a lie down or go to bed, or a favourite teddy etc. When hungry a child may go and get their own plate or dish, or their cup when thirsty. They may know that car keys mean going out for a drive and may take them to their parent/carer when they wish to go out. They may recognise when their blue bag is being packed that they are going to respite for an overnight stay. Again these behaviours will be individual to the child and will develop as they learn.

Makaton

Makaton originated in the 1970s from a communication system for adults with hearing impairments, and has developed from then for use by both children and adults with a variety of communication difficulties. Makaton is a very accessible method of communication and is now used widely in many settings. There are children's TV programmes that use Makaton to help develop sign and communication. There are different topics and it can be used on a basic level, being more simplistic for those children who have severe communication difficulties or for people who have poor memory retention, while a child with greater understanding can use Makaton at a more complex stage having acquired and developed a higher level of skill in its use.

Makaton uses speech alongside signs (gestures) and symbols (pictures) in order to help people communicate their needs, wishes and feelings. Facial expressions, eye contact and body language also give information and help with communication processes, allowing the child to communicate as much information as possible. Makaton should support spoken language and the signs and symbols are used with speech, in spoken word order. Once again, Makaton can be used in a flexible way and be tailored to an individual's needs. It is used in many schools for children with disabilities. If a child is using Makaton, you should encourage the parents and significant adults to learn it to enable effective communication and to reduce frustration and behavioural problems. Makaton is usually used throughout the child's life, hence the many different signs and symbols and stages of complexity as they develop and continue to use Makaton into adulthood.

You may be familiar with Mr Tumble, a favourite for children with and without disabilities. We suggest you see 'Taking it further' for a useful link, and there is also a useful website offering information about classes for parents and other information. You can also look on YouTube for simple Makaton tutorials.

Eye gazers (assistive technology)

An eye gazer is a piece of technology that aids communication, with a control system operated by the eyes. They assist the child with their communication, thus empowering them to be much more independent despite often having severe disabilities that impact upon their ability to communicate and interact with people and their surroundings. The child looks at their controls or cells on a screen and by doing so can generate speech, either by typing a message or using pre-programmed phrases that they are familiar with or use a lot. These systems are being developed as technology improves. You do need to consider that children and young people who use these need time and patience, and they can quickly become tired, particularly if they have complex disabilities that also affect their development and well-being. For example, a child may be non-verbal, have cerebral palsy and epilepsy, which in itself can prove debilitating, and it is likely they will be taking medication that may also make them drowsy or their reaction time much slower.

iPad/tablets

These are great devices for opening up a child's world to communication, interactive games and apps. You can use interactive apps developed to help communication to engage with children and young people of all ages.

My key communication

You can support parents in developing a brief outline of their child's key forms of communication, which could be laminated and become an essential piece of information that they carry with them, especially when visiting new settings with new people. During the getting to know each other period at the beginning of your involvement this would be a useful exercise to help you learn how best to communicate with their child, which would help you build effective communication with the child from an early stage. Here is an example:

Hello, my name is Jonathan but I like it if you call me Jonny.

- » Please look at me directly when speaking to me so that I can see your mouth move, which helps me to know what you are saying.

- » I need you to tap my arm gently to get my attention and to look at you.

- » Please keep your instructions short, with just one instruction at a time. If you give me two things to do I will forget the first one.

- » I am easily distracted by background noises, which make it difficult for me to hear you and to focus, so please think about what other noises are around when you are speaking to me. Try and find a quiet place.

- » Please do not ask me questions about my feelings as I do not understand how to describe these.

Children and young people with a hearing impairment

You will know from your learning around child development and attachment theory that babies start to communicate before they can talk, and to understand and interact with those around them – particularly their significant caregiver. Stimulation is essential to help child development and communication and for understanding of their world – and yours. Babies need visual cues such as eye contact and to read your facial expressions, and also to have the 'cooing' and baby talk – babbling and responses to their babbling. This is no different for a deaf baby – these are all important communication techniques that are a natural part of the development of communication for all children.

Some signs that a child may have a hearing problem:

> » They may shout or talk loudly, or they may speak very softly
>
> » Delayed in his/her speech
>
> » Does not respond to their name when being called
>
> » Complains of not being able to hear you, asks you to repeat things a lot
>
> » Has poor results in reading and oral subjects but good results in other subjects
>
> » Does not contribute in class or in group discussions
>
> » Does not hear things going on nearby or pick up on other conversations
>
> » Does not follow instructions or misunderstands things easily, requiring repeated explanations of what to do before they understand
>
> » Seems to be daydreaming or not paying attention to what's going on
>
> » Misinterprets some words
>
> » Words are not pronounced correctly, or speech is not clear or is slurred.

Routine hearing tests are offered to babies and children to identify any problems early in a child's development, therefore it is hoped that the child should receive early intervention to maximise their hearing. The tests are painless. Some of the following tests may be used:

> » Automated otoacoustic emission (AOAE)
>
> » Automated auditory brainstem response (AABR)
>
> » Visual reinforcement audiometry (VRA)
>
> » Tympanometry
>
> » Conditioned play audiometry (CPA)
>
> » Bone conduction test

» Pure tone audiometry

» Speech perception test

(DfES 2004:60 and www.nhs.uk/Conditions/Hearing-and-vision-tests-
for-children/Pages/Introduction.aspx#children)

Types of hearing loss

There are two main types of deafness – conductive deafness and sensorineural deafness; they can exist in combination. Many deaf children can hear some sounds, and
with modern hearing aids and improved technology deaf children and young people
can often hear more sounds. Deafness can range from mild or moderate to severe
or profound. Unfortunately, not all parents are proactive in learning how to communicate with their deaf child and this can cause many difficulties for both child
and parent(s), including behavioural difficulties being displayed by the child borne
out of frustration that they are not able to communicate many of their basic needs
to the parent/carer. Some parents seem to feel they do not need to learn sign language and that they still know how to communicate with their child. Some think that
because they have 'got by' in the early years they will continue to be able to understand their child. They do not consider that perhaps their child has been able to
understand what is expected of them but as the child grows up, the parents are not
able to understand the growing needs of their child. As the child learns how to use
sign language, perhaps at school, their parents will be left behind and not be able to
enjoy effective communication with their child, for example helping them with their
homework. This can have a detrimental impact on home life and the relationship
between parent and child.

Conductive deafness: it is less common for conductive deafness to be permanent,
and it is often only a temporary hearing loss. Conductive deafness is when sound does
not carry through the outer ear canal into the eardrum and the tiny bones of the middle ear – this may be due to a blockage of ear wax, an ear infection or the presence of
a foreign body. You may have heard of 'glue ear', which is very common in children
under five; this is when the child has fluid in their middle ear. Hearing loss may also be
due to an abnormality in the structure of the middle ear or a ruptured eardrum. Many
types of conductive hearing loss can be corrected by surgery.

Sensorineural deafness is irreversible and is a hearing loss in the inner ear. It is also
referred to as cochlear, sensory, neural or inner hearing loss. Permanent sensorineural
hearing loss is the result of damage within the hearing nerve or to the hair cells within
the cochlea (or both). When the hair cells are damaged they cannot be repaired.

Mixed hearing loss is when conductive hearing loss occurs in combination with sensorineural hearing loss, which can be due to damage in both the inner ear (cochlea) or auditory nerve and the outer or middle ear.

There are lots of support groups available, many online, that you can direct parents to. The Royal National Institute for Deaf People (RNID) www.rnid.org.uk or The National Deaf Children's Society www.ndcs.org.uk are good starting points. Parents should be given support at diagnosis, where they are likely to be referred to their local education service who will give information about how to proceed with getting the right support and education for their child.

Methods for assisting communication for hearing-impaired children

Listening and learning is an important skill for a deaf child, and their development will depend on a number of factors, such as how deaf they are, when the deafness was identified, when hearing aids were introduced and how well they work for the child. Professionals will facilitate a deaf child's development and continue to support and monitor the child throughout each stage of their development, helping with their communicative development, interaction and play. They will advise about different expectations as to how the child should develop and achieve, how parents should respond to their child's needs and what adaptations are appropriate and at what stage. There are developmental checklists that identify detailed profiles for the milestones a child should achieve (DfES 2004).

British Sign Language (BSL): Not all deaf children and young people use BSL – some will use speech or will combine both methods (known as sign bilingualism), when a child is encouraged to use the spoken word and a sign language at the same time. There are many children who do not have English as a first language, so their parents may use their native tongue. Communication may therefore be in spoken form with signs taken from BSL (known as Sign Supported English, SSE). It is important to ascertain how the child prefers to communicate. See British Deaf Association: www.bda.org.uk.

Total Communication (TC): TC involves selecting the most appropriate method of communication for the deaf child, with sign being used as a support to oral communication to enable the child's remaining hearing to be maximised as a way of helping to develop speech and language skills. Signed English (SE), or SSE, uses signs from BSL and finger spelling. Finger spelling gives each letter of the alphabet its own sign and is used particularly when signing names of words that do not have a sign.

Here are a few helpful things to consider when communicating with children and young people who are deaf:

- » Good eye contact – look at the child straight on.

- » Speak normally – don't talk slowly just because the child can't hear you, and don't shout: deaf children may be able to lipread so you need to speak naturally and not cover your mouth when talking.

- » Don't all talk at once – if there are several people together there may be two conversations going on at once, which would be very difficult for a deaf child to follow.

- » Use visual clues – if telling someone it's time to go, for example, point to your watch or the door.

- » Don't keep changing the topic of conversation without telling the child.

- » Ensure that background noise is limited.

- » Good lighting – important for reading the speaker's face and lipreading, and seeing a child's facial expressions clearly.

- » Ensure the child's hearing aids are comfortable and fit properly.

- » Tiredness – a deaf child has to try harder to hear and may become tired more quickly than other children. This may lead to frustration and behavioural issues if they are misunderstood.

- » Give information in small chunks to avoid overload.

A child or young person may find it useful to have additional support, such as Cued Speech. This is a lipreading supplement that uses eight hand shapes in four different positions near the mouth while speaking. This should be done while the child is looking at you.

Types of hearing aids/technology to support communication

Hearing aids: there are different types of hearing aids and it is important that parents seek the best advice for their child's individual needs. Children who are introduced to hearing aids from a very young age are more likely to accept them. Technology is changing and improving all the time and there are more devices being introduced that are implanted in the skull (bone anchored) with an external abutment and detachable sound processor.

Cochlear implants are electronic devices that are surgically implanted into the inner ear (or cochlea) to provide sound signals to the brain for a person who is moderately to profoundly deaf. The implant does the work that the damaged cochlea is not doing. Some people may have bilateral cochlear implants, ie in both ears.

Radio aid: some deaf children may wear a radio aid system together with hearing aids or cochlear implants. Radio aids have two main parts, a transmitter and a receiver. A 'Soundfield' system is often used in schools.

Please see the National Deaf Children's Society website for more information on technology for deaf children: www.ndcs.org.uk.

Children and young people with a visual impairment

The eye is the most developed organ of the body at birth and it develops more quickly than any other immediately after birth. Despite vision being poor when first born, at three weeks of age the eye is one of the most active parts of the body. A child's vision normally develops most during the first four to six months and then during the first year, so by their first birthday babies have usually developed a wide range of visual skills. Vision continues to develop up to the age of seven, when it has reached its maturity. Forty percent of the brain is devoted to processing visual information, which it associates with that received from the other senses – touch, hearing, smell, taste and our position in space (DfES 2004a).

When a person's sight is not developed correctly they may be said to be partially sighted, have low vision or sight loss or be blind – these terms could be described collectively as having a visual impairment. Serious loss of vision in childhood is rare and often children can see something, even if this is limited and may only be light and dark images. Children with more mild visual loss, unilateral visual problems or eye disease without visual consequences are more common.

It is sometimes difficult to establish why a child has a visual impairment. Vision must be stimulated to reach its full potential and also requires good perceptual skills in order to make sense of the images that are sent to the brain from the eye. Because of this, it is often only later in a child's development that the full extent of their visual impairment becomes apparent. Undetected eye problems can seriously affect a child's development intellectually, socially and physically. Visual problems are also associated with other disabilities, such as Down's syndrome and cerebral palsy.

Sight tests are free for children up to 16 years of age. A child's vision can be screened, which is an efficient and cost-effective way to identify children with visual impairments or eye conditions that are likely to lead to a visual impairment. There are a number of methods that can be chosen to screen the child, dependent upon their age (see www.patient.info/doctor/Vision-Testing-and-Screening-in-Young-Children.htm).

Some common significant eye problems for children are:

Strabismus (squint) – the most common cause of amblyopia, an incorrect alignment of the eyes as a result of physical obstruction to eye movement or injury or disease affecting the eye muscle or nerve supplying the muscles.

Amblyopia (lazy eye) – a result of a defect that is present in infancy or early years, preventing the eye from receiving adequate stimulation and causing a reduction in vision

Defective binocular vision – is a consequence of a squint or amblyopia and is the inability to use the two eyes together correctly, leading to depth perception impairment.

Hypermetropia (long-sightedness) and **myopia (short-sightedness)** can affect older children.

Remember a child may not always say (or be able to say) if they are having trouble with their eyes. Because visual problems are not normally painful, the child may not recognise there is anything wrong.

Indications that a child may have eye problems:

» Rubbing their eyes a lot (when they are not tired)

» Excessively watery eyes

» Screwing up an eye or closing it when watching television or reading, or sitting very close to the television

» Reluctant to join in activities such as drawing or reading or when close work is involved

» Poor hand–eye co-ordination and clumsiness

» Unexplained headaches

» White reflection glimmer in the eye

» A squint or lazy eye – they are often hereditary but not always obvious

» Blurred or double vision

»   Difficulty walking on uneven surfaces

»   At a few months old a baby's eyes should be able to follow you around a room. Briefly cover each eye in turn and if the baby dislikes one eye being covered more than the other there may be a problem.

(www.lookafteryoureyes.org/eye-care/children/stages-of-development/)

Communication and visually impaired children

When a child is born with a visual impairment there is no doubt that this will have immediate effects upon their communication. As discussed with hearing impaired children, from birth babies learn from their significant carers and focusing on their faces will open up communication. The baby looks at their mother or father (or significant carer), they respond and engage with the baby, the baby reciprocates etc, and thus the attachment process develops. A child who has a visual impairment will not be able to respond in the same way. They do not pick up the signals and thus the carer does not respond in the same way. The child may not give eye contact, or this may be much less frequently than a child without a visual impairment. The baby may not develop responses such as smiles and babbling at the same rate, if at all, and the development of communication is delayed. The child may be much more passive and not notice what is going on around them or take an active interest, for example at someone nearby, bright colours, glistening sunlight or reflections, which in turn means they are not communicating what is going on around them and their feelings and emotions about their own world. A natural progression would be for a child to see something, look at it and give cues that they were interested, so the caregiver would respond, for example the child looks at a colourful ball, the parent will give the ball to the child and they will play together. This also encourages vocal sounds and babbling and so on. Some children with a visual impairment may have additional learning difficulties or other sensory impairments, which compound their development even further, as would multiple disabilities (RNIB 2011).

Some children with complex needs and visual impairments will require 'alternative augmentative communication' (AAC). Those working with children with communication difficulties will often augment their spoken language to help the child to understand and develop spoken language skills. Children who have not developed speech correctly, have no speech or are unable to use symbols for communication will require alternative ways to express their themselves (RNIB 2011). There is no 'one size fits all' method of communication and different children will require different methods.

These could include visual aids, including pictures and symbols of different textures and materials, and voice-output communication aids.

Some fun ways to help develop language and communication in a child with a visual impairment are listed below. Use the tips already discussed in this chapter and remember to have fun and where possible make the interactions a happy time for the child or young person, allowing them to feel comfortable. Break down the barriers.

> » Play naming games – use an object as a toy and say the name of the object, name the spoon when feeding/eating etc.

> » Give clear commentary about what is happening and going on around them. This helps blind babies and children feel secure and understand their environment, and will encourage communication.

> » Provide children with brightly coloured toys and a plain contrasting background, and use coloured lights and torches in play.

> » Praise the child each time they use language, use repetitive nursery rhymes and songs and do actions with the songs, do sing-a-longs.

> » Looking in the mirror, wear wigs, hats and beards and let the child feel textures of the beard etc.

> » Water games – using squirty washing-up bottles and water play or playing with bubbles.

> » Sensory rooms – with lights and bubble machines, soft play materials and crash mats, wind machines and music. Parents could convert a room if they have space – it doesn't have to be too costly (also good for hearing impaired).

There are lots of things that parents will need to consider and that you will need to think about when working with children with visual impairments – you can get advice from the other professionals involved and at meetings such as school reviews, Child in Need meetings, from family (the real expert on their child) and from The Royal National Institute of Blind People (RNIB) charity. You can direct parents to the RNIB email helpline, and advise that they request a referral to the Sight Loss Counselling Team (RNIB and Action For Blind People working together). They can be contacted through TypeTalk in the same way.

Braille – Some children may wish to learn braille (or Moon) as an alternative to traditional print. Braille is a tactile form of reading made up of raised dots that form letters and words. Children learn using a braille machine known as a Perkins Brailler, which has six keys that make the raised dots on special paper (DfES 2004a: 61).

Moon is another form of raised lines and curves that create basic shapes, which is said to be easier to learn than braille; some letters resemble the print equivalent. Some children with additional physical and/or learning difficulties can acquire some literacy skills through learning Moon (www.rnib.org.uk).

Written information

For those who are partially sighted and can read text and written information there are a few things to consider: you may need to use both words and pictures and have text that is much larger so they can read it. You need to ensure you use short, clear sentences in simple language, correctly coloured paper, words not abbreviations, full stops and bullet points, active verbs and bold to highlight important words. Consider using DVDs or CDs to support written information.

Deaf-blind

On top of all the issues discussed above, there are extra considerations to be made when communicating with or supporting a deaf-blind child. A deaf-blind child will not hear you trying to describe what you're about to do or be able to see you approach them, which means there is a risk that they can be shocked or surprised by how you first make your presence known to them. The child needs to have a gentle touch on their hand only to begin with so that they can be aware that you are there and are going to communicate with them. Objects of reference are a good way to let the child know what is happening next or where they are being taken. For example, to place a sponge or flannel in their hand would let them know it is wash or bath time. Placing the child's hands on your throat as you speak would help them feel the vibration of your voice, which gives them a sensory experience. These are just a few ideas and there are specialist organisations that provide training opportunities to develop this level of communication. Sense is a national charity supporting and campaigning for people who are deaf-blind and those with sensory impairments. For further information, see www.sense.org.uk.

Dyslexia

Dyslexia is a learning difficulty that can affect a child's ability to learn and do reading and writing, although it does not usually affect intelligence. You may recognise that a child has dyslexia if they read and write slowly, write letters the wrong way around and confuse 'd' and 'b' etc, are inconsistent with their spelling, are unable to follow sequences when given instructions or struggle to plan and organise things.

There are charities that offer support, such as Dyslexia Action www.dyslexiaaction. org.uk/ and the British Dyslexia Association (BDA) www.bdadyslexia.org.uk/.

Dyspraxia (developmental co-ordination disorder)

Children with dyspraxia may be delayed in meeting their milestones and take longer to achieve rolling over, sitting, crawling or walking. As they begin to walk they may be stiff (hypertonia) or floppy (hypotonia) and have co-ordination difficulties. Other difficulties you may notice include:

» saying some words and putting sentences together

» catching a ball or playing team sports

» gross and fine motor skills

» writing – illegible handwriting and cannot copy off the board

» holding a pen or cutlery

» struggling to co-ordinate muscle movements in their mouth (apraxia)

» using a phone – texting or using a keyboard

» bumping into things, falling over and struggling with balance, being clumsy

In addition to this a child with dyspraxia may have difficulty concentrating and a short attention span. They cannot follow instructions or copy information down and this may become more noticeable when they are in school – perhaps they may not do homework because they have not been able to write it down, and they are therefore thought to be lazy or just troublesome. They may be slow to learn new skills and also have difficulty with friendships and low self-esteem – perhaps linked to how they are perceived by other people. Children with dyspraxia may not have a problem with intelligence and despite their difficulties their abilities to think, talk and understand are not usually behind what is expected at his or her age. As with dyslexia the SENCO can help put support in place and further assessment can be completed by educational psychologists.

(www.nhs.uk/conditions/dyspraxia-(childhood)/Pages/Symptoms.aspx)

We hope you have found this chapter to be informative and that it has given you some food for thought about how to communicate with children who have a disability. Finally, we would like to remind you about the Mental Capacity Act and how communication links to this.

Mental Capacity Act and communication

In Chapter 1, we discussed the Mental Capacity Act and how it is important to assume a person has the capacity to make decisions in their lives. In order to do this, you may need to look at the different methods discussed in this chapter that are available to enhance your communication with young adults with communication difficulties to help you assess their capacity, advocate on their behalf and make their voices heard. There are five key principles for considering a person's mental capacity and these ALL require good communication skills:

» Assume person has capacity

» Support the person to make their decision

» Unwise decision making is OK, *if* they have all the information they need to make their choice – you don't have to agree with their decision

» You must act in the person's best interest

» Choose less restrictive options – any intervention should be weighed against individual circumstances.

Finally, a reminder of why communication is important for all children. Article 12 of the UN Convention on the Rights of the Child states, '*Respect the views of the child*' (UNICEF 2012). This means that every child has the right to say what they think regarding all matters affecting them, and to have their views taken seriously. It is your responsibility, in your role as their social worker therefore, to ensure children are listened to and that their views are central to the work that you do both *with* and *on behalf of* all children and young people.

Taking it further

Gully, T (2014) *The Critical Years: Early Years Development from Conception to 5*. Critical Publishing – Chapters 2 to 4 inclusive

First Steps – A guide for parents of children with visual impairments on medical terms, eye conditions, key professionals and services available. Revised Edition ED289 [Print] and ED293 [Disk] – RNIB publication

Which Way? – For parents of children with visual impairments and additional complex communication, learning or physical disabilities – this complements the First Steps publication above. RNIB Publication Revised Edition ED296 [Print] ED297 [Disk]

Free website for communication resources:

Giving Greetings – www.givinggreetings.com/freestuff.html

Makaton – www.makaton.org/aboutMakaton/ and a great website showing you how to use Makaton: www.bbc.co.uk/cbeebies/grownups/makaton

Chapter 5 | Autism and its impact on communication

Within this chapter we discuss autism and the autistic spectrum, including Asperger's syndrome. We have chosen to look at autism in more detail than other disabilities because there are an increasing number of children and young people on caseloads who have autism or traits of autistic spectrum disorders (ASD) and we felt it important that you have some understanding about how autism affects communication. We will take a look at the areas of the brain affected by autism, the 'triad of impairments' and hypo- and hyper-sensitivity. We discover communication from the perspective of a child with autism using PECS and schedules, with an example of how it supports autistic children to use visual timetables to help with their communication.

The work of Leo Kanner (1943) and Hans Asperger (1944) forms the basis of today's understanding and knowledge about ASD. Here we will touch on the basics in order to give you some understanding of a child with ASD, how they see the world and what it is like within their world. We hope that by helping you understand a little more about the complexities of autism, and how it affects a child's communication, it will help give you some ideas to think about why a child may or may not communicate and behave in a certain way. We advise you to do your own research about autistic spectrum and associated disorders depending upon how much you wish or need to know on this very interesting topic.

A child with severe autism may present as:

» Plays alone, is disinterested in others and the world around them – no imaginary play

» No or limited verbal communication, possibly echolalia

» Having challenging behaviours due to frustration, often borne out of difficulties in their communication

» Self-harming

» No or only brief eye contact

» Appears to be 'in their own world'

» Unable to form relationships (even with close family)

» Little or no empathy or not want to hug or be close to others/avoidant

» Poor motor skills

» Fiddling with objects, body rocking, finger flicking etc.

» Likes routine and everything to be the same all the time – shows behavioural problems when there is even the slightest change in any routine

» Lines up objects, develops obsessions

» Has sensory difficulties – doesn't like loud noises or strong smells, or possibly vice versa, sensory processing difficulties, over-reaction to textures, certain foods etc.

Autism Act 2009

There is now more awareness about autism. The Autism Act 2009 gained royal assent on 12 November 2009 and makes provision for meeting the needs of adults with autistic spectrum conditions, and for connected purposes. It was followed by the 'autism strategy', published in 2010 and updated in 2014 – *Think Autism: Fulfilling and Rewarding Lives, the strategy for adults with autism in England: an update.* In 2015, further guidance was published, *Statutory guidance for Local Authorities and NHS organisations to support implementation of the Adult Autism Strategy.* Although primarily for adults, the guidance does (in Chapter 3, p 22) discuss the importance of planning in relation to young people with autism and their transition to adulthood, and mentions recent legislation like the Care Act 2014 and the Children and Families Act 2014, including SEND.

What is autism?

The term autism is also used as an umbrella term for autistic spectrum conditions, including Asperger's syndrome. Within this section when we discuss autism or Asperger's and associated difficulties and any strategies, we are talking about children and not adults; however, many of the difficulties presented will be the same for adults and children. We hope that nobody is offended by the terminology used within this chapter.

Autism is a lifelong condition and it is estimated that there are more than 500,000 people in England on the autism spectrum, including those with high functioning Asperger's syndrome (Social Care et al 2015a:3). According to the National Autistic Society (NAS), there is strong evidence to suggest that autism can be caused by a variety of environmental or neurological factors, all of which affect brain development. There is also evidence to suggest genetic factors are responsible for some forms of autism, but it is not a result of poor parenting. This does not mean that a child will 'acquire' autism but there may be a trigger or an associated condition, eg a learning disability, Fragile X, epilepsy, Down's syndrome, a birth trauma or prolonged pregnancy.

An autism diagnosis is relatively rare in girls; Asperger's is even rarer. Boys outnumber girls with autism by four to one; in 'high-functioning autism' and Asperger's the gender ratio is estimated to be 10:1 (Dworzynski et al 2012).

Autistic spectrum conditions are also known as pervasive development disorders (PDD), the more well-known being autism and Asperger's. There are also:

» Deficits in attention and motor perception (DAMP)

» DAMP combined with ADHD

» Developmental co-ordination disorder (DCD, or dyspraxia)

In some circumstances a person may not meet specific criteria for autism or Asperger's but present with symptoms of ADHD and/or DCD and will often be diagnosed as having a PDD.

Diagnosis

Autism may be diagnosed in the child's early years (2–3 years old) when it is becoming more noticeable that they are not meeting their milestones. There may be delayed development in certain areas, the child pays less attention to others and the world around them, or their behaviours are seen as 'different', ie not in line with that of their peers. For example, a toddler of 12–18 months would usually be bringing a toy to you to engage in play, making eye contact and pointing at things, but a child with autism may not do this and instead seem to be in their own little world. Autism is not always identified early on, however, and may not be diagnosed until the child is attending an educational setting, when it becomes clearer that they are not meeting their milestones. Some children with autism may not have an Education, Health and Care Plan (EHC) (the old Statement of Educational Need) (see Chapter 1 for the EHC process), particularly if they are high-functioning, and might remain in a mainstream setting, while other children with more severe needs may go on to have an EHC plan and be educated within a special school.

A diagnosis of autism is a medical decision and usually involves professional input from the Community Paediatric Team – speech, language and occupational therapists, child psychiatrist and clinical and/or child psychologist – who will undertake detailed observations of the child in different settings, such as home and school, detailed assessments including developmental history and functioning, gather details of prenatal, family history and other health issues, and also use specific tools (such as Conners' questionnaire) in order to make their diagnosis (NICE 2011). Having a diagnosis can offer some relief to many parents as it explains their child's behaviour and why they are presenting differently to their peers. A diagnosis may also give access to useful resources, for example specific parenting courses, support groups and services in educational settings and health and social care or universal/voluntary groups in the community. This can also offer parents contact with other parents who are adapting to life with a child with autism and the grief and loss they often experience when coming to terms with a diagnosis (see Chapter 3).

The functions of the brain typically affected by autism

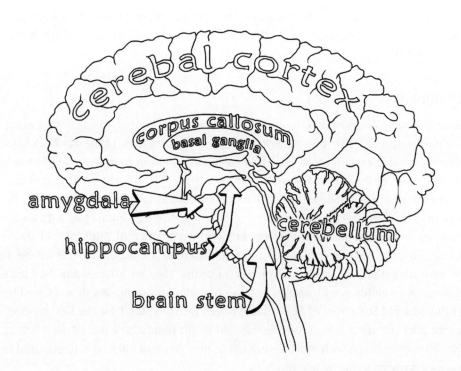

The Brain Box (what does what in our brains?)		
The *amygdala* [emotional centre] • responsible for basic survival skills such as emotions and social behaviour including fear, anger and sex.	The *basal ganglia* • control automatic movement • cluster of structures in the centre of the brain (central hemisphere) connecting the cerebrum and cerebellum	The *cerebellum* [means little brain] • found at the rear of the brain at the top of the brain stem • important for 'fine motor' activity and balance, coordination, which muscles you would use and your body movements (skilled movements/ learning pathways).
The *cerebral cortex* • controls most of the bodily functions • responsible for general movement, perception and behavioural responses • memories are stored and retrieved from here • consists of thin layer of gray matter on the surface of the cerebrum	The *corpus callosum* • connects the left and right hemispheres of the brain, facilitating communication between them	The *hippocampus* • processes new information for long-term storage and memory of recent events • supports navigation and spatial awareness • without this you would forget what you did today – only remembering old memories
The *brain stem* • situated at the front of the cerebellum and sends messages to different parts of the body and the cerebral cortex • controls (survival instinct) automatic responses and functions – heart rate, blood pressure, breathing, sleep, reflexes, limb movements, digestion and urination (visceral functions) • connected to the spinal cord		

The earlier the brain function is altered the more severe the autism is likely to be. Any effect in pregnancy is likely to be more severe as the baby's brain is not yet fully developed. There are irregularities in the brain structures themselves in the areas shown in the diagram, such as in the corpus callosum, amygdala and cerebellum. It is believed that these abnormalities occur during prenatal development. In addition, there are imbalances in neurotransmitters – chemicals that help nerve cells communicate with one another. Two of the neurotransmitters that appear to be affected are serotonin (which affects emotion and behaviour) and glutamate (which plays a role in neuron activity). Together, these brain differences may account for autistic behaviour.

For more information see www.health.howstuffworks.com/mental-health/autism/autism3.htm.

Early in childhood, the brains of autistic children grow faster and larger than those of children without autism. Later, when the brains of children without autism get bigger and better organised, autistic children's brains grow more slowly. An autistic brain is 'wired' differently and information is not communicated properly.

The spectrum

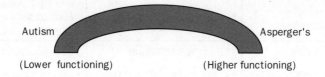

Autism   Asperger's

(Lower functioning)   (Higher functioning)

People with ASD, as the term suggests, are often viewed as being on a spectrum from very low-functioning to very high-functioning. Those on the lower end of the spectrum are normally diagnosed with autistic disorder (autism) due to their severe symptoms, and they function much lower in most areas of their lives, often being unable to live independently. Those on the high end of the spectrum are considered to have Asperger's or AD with mild symptoms, functioning relatively well and often living independent adult lives. Children (and adults) who are on the spectrum may present with traits that are interlinked from both Asperger's and autism and therefore at times you may not easily recognise where they fit; when people are referred to as being 'on the spectrum' they may fall somewhere inbetween these two states.

A child with autism would have restricted interests and repetitive behaviours. Communication is greatly impaired for many, and some are non-verbal or have very limited verbal communication. Those with Asperger's syndrome are often of average or above average intelligence. They have fewer problems with speech but may still have difficulties with understanding and processing language. Despite functioning at a higher level, they do demonstrate some features of the triad of impairments (discussed below).

Recent studies have shown that approximately 70% of people with autism also meet diagnostic criteria for at least one other (often unrecognised) psychiatric disorder that is further impairing their psychosocial functioning. Intellectual disability (intelligence quotient [IQ] below 70) occurs in approximately 50% of young people with autism. (NICE 2011:128)

The triad of impairments

Lorna Wing and Judith Gould (1979) contributed greatly to the understanding of autism and concluded that social impairment is a disorder of development that shows across all areas of the spectrum of related disorders. They identified three areas of development forming a cluster of features that provide diagnostic criteria for the identification of autism, known as the triad of impairments:

» difficulty with social communication;

» difficulty with social interaction;

» difficulty with social understanding and imagination.

Difficulty with social communication

The processing of information can be slowed down significantly in autism. Think about when you use a computer and the internet connection is slow and it keeps searching for the website you want, or you are typing and the computer is not showing your text on screen because you are typing too fast. These are processing problems, which are what happens in the autistic brain.

A baby has no verbal communication and uses 'babble', smiling and crying to communicate. As they develop they begin to show what they want by other behaviours that become their main method of communication until their speech takes over. For example, a three-year-old would have a vocabulary of several hundred words and this would keep increasing as their communication skills develop; because they have a large bank of words for communication, their dependency on other behaviours will decrease.

An autistic child's language and communication does not develop at the same rate, and they may only have three words. They are more reliant on their behaviour as a method of communication and they may have learnt more behaviour to express their needs, to replace verbal communication. This behaviour, however, is imprecise compared with language. A child with autism may have learnt to lead by the hand to the cupboard to show that they want a biscuit as they cannot just say this.

Communication is a complex area for children (and adults) with autism. Some develop their own language or have some word variation, with unusual patterns of communication due to the difficulty in processing information. They may process information more slowly and need a long time to answer, or they may be very fast. You may notice some children will repeat the last word they hear (this is known as echolalia) and others may speak in the third person, which is known as pronominal reversal. An autistic child's tone of voice may be inappropriate to what they are saying. They may sound excited but actually be afraid and not sure how to say something. Remember that a child may say more than they understand or understand more than they can say, and that children who are non-verbal may fully understand you while other children may not have an understanding of the words but still speak them. As discussed in this chapter, a child may understand the words but not be able to process the information in a sentence. Saying a long sentence like 'Get your coat on because we are going out; I will wait in the car' would be too much for them to process, but they may understand key words such as coat, out and car.

A child with Asperger's syndrome may speak fluently, but other children who are on the spectrum have difficulty with their communication skills. Problems can include:

» Difficulty in reading facial expressions and body language or interpreting the differences in tone of voice – processing language and differentiating between words that sound the same but have different meanings.

» Difficulty in understanding spoken words and metaphors/sarcasm – they take things literally. Many autistic children have a literal understanding. For example, think about a discussion between a parent and child with the parent telling their child 'pull your socks up' to express the need for them to behave better; to an autistic child this would literally be understood as their parent wanting them to pull their socks up in the physical sense. Or a parent asks their autistic child to 'wait a minute' only to find that the child literally counts to 60 (if able to) and then comes back expecting to have their parent's full attention.

» Some parents who do not fully understand these behaviours as part of their child's make-up may see their child as defiant or sarcastic. The child will not understand why his actions or words are making his parents angry.

» Difficulty following simple instructions and complicated sentences – they can only follow one-word instructions (see Chapter 7 for further information and an activity about giving instructions). A child with Asperger's may also have difficulty with this aspect of communication despite having a higher level of verbal communication.

A child with autism would not necessarily understand that language is a tool that is used to share information with another person, would not talk about their feelings or maybe even understand them, and would not understand the emotions of others.

Difficulty with social interaction (relationships)

A young person may appear to be withdrawn and uninterested in what is going on around them and in other people. A young person with autism would have difficulty with meeting people and forming social relationships. There is a difference in that a child or young person with Asperger's would still have these difficulties but be more *aware* that they had them and thus manage them better. A young person with autism would have difficulty reading another person's body language and would not pick up on social cues. They would not know possibly that if a person was crossing their arms they may be stand-offish, or if they are yawning and looking around the room that they are bored and not listening to them. They would also not show an interest in other people or empathise with them if they were upset. They may pass you a tissue if you are crying but only because they have learnt that this is what someone does when a person starts to cry rather than actually empathising with why you are upset and crying. Sometimes their behaviours can be seen as rude by others because they don't have the skills to fit in socially, and they may stand out in a group. The young person may laugh when it is inappropriate or smile at the wrong time etc.

Some young people with autism may not like physical contact whereas others may enjoy different types of physical contact – perhaps really tight hugs or blankets around them. There are weighted blankets or weighted backpacks to help the child feel secure and meet their sensory needs (you may want to look up sensory diets). An autistic child is less likely to seek out a hug from parents or they may do things that are repetitive or in a certain way, and they are done to meet their needs rather than anyone else's, ie when they want a hug they will have one, but they are less likely to pay attention when someone else may want one.

Another reason why many children with high-functioning autism and Asperger's have difficulties with social relationships and situations could be because they have problems with facial recognition – AKA 'face blindness' or its technical names of prosopagnosia or facial agnosia. Until a relationship is well established many children with facial blindness may struggle to recognise a new classmate as they do not remember their facial features; when they see the child in class they may not recognise them as the person they were with the day before. It is rare, however, that they do not recognise and become familiar with that person once they know them well, but it can be difficult and create barriers to forming/building new relationships (see – www.myaspergerchild.com).

Difficulty with social imagination and understanding

A child with autism will often have repetitive behaviours and 'rituals' and they lack imagination. Some children may show a range of behaviours, such as:

» Self-harm, seeking the sensory stimulation

» Aversion to loud noises or seeking them out, or not liking bright lights. Often they may hear noises that we would ordinarily not be aware of, such as a slight humming noise from a radio or television

» Turning lights on and off, closing doors or putting chairs under tables

» Developing different rituals and obsessions that last a long time, for example they may go to the train station all the time, know everything about lots of types of trains, train timetables etc

» Not being able to tell a lie – they follow rules very strictly

» Only eating certain foods – perhaps those of a particular colour or texture.

The child may exhibit behaviour such as walking on their tip toes, flapping their arms, jumping up and down or spinning around. They may have difficulty with games and co-ordination. Many autistic children do not like change.

Scenario: Abid and the road works

Abid is 12 years old and has learning difficulties and autism. He goes to a school that is ten miles away from his home. Abid is collected on school transport (a taxi) from home and taken to school with an escort, and he returns home on the same transport. Abid has to follow a certain routine every morning before the taxi arrives. Abid's taxi arrives at 8.05am each morning and it normally takes 20 minutes to get to school; he is collected at 3.10pm for his return journey.

One morning Abid's taxi collected him as usual but Abid became distressed during his journey to school. He began hitting his face and kicking the seat in front of him. When he arrived at school Abid's behaviour steadily deteriorated to the point where he could not remain in his classroom that morning. He did begin to settle after lunchtime and was fine for the rest of the day. On his return home Abid was settled. On the next two days, Abid's behaviour was the same, again not settling down until after lunch, but he was fine on his way home. The school teacher informed Abid's mother about his change in behaviour and on the third day, his mother spoke to the escort. The escort could not understand what the problem was.

On the fourth day, Abid was fine and he settled back into his routine and was also settled at school. Abid's mother again spoke to the escort and it was not until they were talking in more detail and the escort said that they had taken a short diversion via a different street due to road works that Abid's mother was able to understand why he had acted in that way. On the fourth day, the diversion had gone, Abid's route was his usual route and he was once again settled and his problem behaviours stopped. On Abid's return journey the roadworks had been able to allow traffic that was travelling down the road on the right as normal and it was only the traffic travelling in the opposite direction that had been diverted, hence why Abid was only displaying difficult behaviour on the way to school.

Challenging behaviour and meltdowns

You may have heard the term challenging behaviour being used when a child is displaying negative behaviour such as hitting, kicking, screeching loudly, self-harming or continually repeating certain actions. This is called challenging behaviour in that it is difficult for the parent or carer to manage, and the behaviour could be frequent or severe and may impact upon the child within the community or restrict their access to the community. Remember however, what is seen as challenging for one person to cope with may not be for another – it depends on the person having to manage the behaviour, who is being tested by the child's actions. As the child's behaviour escalates, perhaps because they are not able to do what they want to do, maybe one of their rituals, this could then progress into what we call a meltdown: sensory, emotional and information overload – too many demands that are too complex to cope with. Parents often find it draining to manage the child's repetitive behaviour, ie the need to carry out their rituals and the ensuing meltdown if this is not possible. When a child has escalating behaviours or a meltdown you need to think about what the child is trying to communicate through their behaviour. It has a purpose for them and because of their sensory processing/communication difficulties (ie the triad of impairments) they have learnt to communicate through this behaviour: it has become a function and perhaps they have learnt that it will get them their desired outcome. For example, Johnny does not like it when his brother sits next to him on the sofa when he is watching Thomas the Tank Engine on DVD (on repeat as this is his obsession). He does not know how to say 'Go away and leave me alone', but has learnt that when he hits his brother, eventually his brother becomes fed up of this, moves away and Johnny is left to watch his DVD on his own. This is Johnny's way of communicating his wishes. It is not always that simple but you need to think about the presenting behaviour, the hitting, which is the bit you can see, and then you need to think about what is going on with the child that might cause that behaviour – the bit you can't see. This has been likened to the iceberg effect: you can only see a small part of what is going on (above the surface) and you cannot see what is going on underneath – the cause.

It is important to look at how parents can stop the behaviour by helping them think about what may be causing it. We are not going to pretend this is easy, but some of the things within this chapter will give you food for thought, eg the environment may be causing the child to feel sensory overload. While you may be trying to work out what it is that is causing the behaviour, it may be that one behaviour is replaced by another until the actual cause is identified and remedied. When supporting a parent to manage their child who has reached meltdown you need to help them think about the events or triggers preceding the meltdown (some triggers are not easy to see and the child's behaviour may just reach boiling point very quickly) and what they can do to divert the child's behaviour that will satisfy the child's desires/needs or reduce their stress before meltdown occurs. At the same time the parents need to think about themselves and what causes their anxiety to rise, because as the child's behaviour begins to escalate this is likely to increase the parents' apprehension and stress and they too could reach crisis or meltdown. Talk with parents about how they recognise their own and each other's trigger points so they can work to support each other and thus effectively manage their child's behaviours. If dealing with a single parent you may need to ask them about their support networks and how they could utilise these at peak times.

Using a 'low arousal' approach is a positive technique that parents can adopt. This may be difficult at first as it means that they have to stay calm and not respond when Johnny is hitting, kicking and displaying the challenging behaviour and this will be very difficult to do. It is important that the parent/carer who is putting the approach into practice has belief in, and values, what they are doing because combined these traits influence how we respond in different situations. In this example, they need to believe that the change from the negative behaviour will occur and that they are prepared to work to see it through as often this is not a quick fix approach. The low arousal approach focuses on intervention such as decreasing demands and requests to avoid conflict, and avoidance of aggressive responses, for example not standing in a hostile stance toward the young person or avoiding direct eye contact, which can be seen as antagonistic or challenging. Parents or carers may find this difficult as it involves changing their own responses and reflecting upon how they would usually react. Reducing confrontation and putting strategies in place, perhaps using structures, PECS and redirection of behaviour at key times, can reduce outbursts and stress for both parent and child (adapted from Salmon 2015). See www.autism.org.uk for information about preparing a 'meltdown plan' (also see 'Taking it further' below and Chapter 7 for further help on managing behaviour).

Hypo- and hyper-sensitivity

Stephen Shore (2004), himself on the autistic spectrum, has written about sensory integration dysfunction, which means that people on the spectrum perceive the world differently, with some of their senses being turned either too high or too low and the information received through their senses being distorted. Some or all of the five senses (taste, smell, hearing, touch and sight) are said to be hyper- or hypo-sensitive. Shore adds that autistic people do not always recognise proprioceptive and other inner senses. Grandin (1995) also discusses how autistic people have difficulties with their sensory integration – see 'Taking it further' for this text.

Vestibular and proprioceptive senses (in other words, all the receptors, eg our body movement, balance, body positioning, sight (visual), touch, hearing (auditory) and taste) come to the front and our brain sorts out the senses we need at the time to suit what we are doing (www.cherringtonsawers.com/tactile-vestibular-and-proprioceptive-senses.html). If you think of your brain as the main office for all deliveries and messages you receive, you have a 'receptionist' in your brain who sorts out your senses and deals with them as you need them, putting away the ones you do not want to use now (until you need them later), and selecting the ones you want. An autistic child cannot manage all their senses at any one time and becomes overloaded, confused and agitated. Or perhaps the opposite may happen – they have no senses and are withdrawn, or have no responses and are in a catatonic state.

An autistic child may only have one sense as a primary sense rather than both sight and sound. They may recognise someone by smell alone. They would respond to one sense over another, and do not have the ability to decide which senses are needed for which situations.

Examples of sensory problems creating barriers to communication for an autistic child

A child may not be hyper- or hypo-sensitive all the time. We have interpreted www.autism.com/symptoms_sensory_overview and Shore's (2004) points (using our own experience of children with ASD) about sensory difficulties as follows:

Sight (visually)

Hyper-sensitive – finds lights too bright. Fluorescent tubes flicker many times per second; most people cannot see, this but a person who is hyper-sensitive often cannot cope with it. They may sit in the dark to avoid light.

Hypo-sensitive – the brain sees things too darkly. People with hypo-sensitive vision may often look out of the corner of their eye, using their peripheral vision. The child may appear clumsy as they do not see things because they appear dark, and they may want the lights on all the time. In school an autistic child may want to sit near the window but their teacher thinks this is too distracting for them and moves them away from the window without realising that it is the light they are seeking; this may result in a tantrum.

Hearing (auditory)

Hyper-sensitive – autistic children may hear the slightest sound and can hear lots of conversations at once but cannot filter the information received. They become overwhelmed and may wear ear defenders. They may hear a fridge buzzing or the boiler, kettle or fan in the oven, so they do not listen to what you are saying as these other noises dominate their concentration.

Hypo-sensitive – the child does not hear well; things may be more muffled but they are not deaf. They cannot work out what is being said. They may have the television or their music at high volume and they seek noises, yet they may be troubled by other noises that are unpredictable, eg a dog barking, an alarm going off or a telephone ringing.

Touch (tactile)

Hyper-sensitive – an autistic child may avoid certain fabrics such as wool and want to only wear cotton. They would avoid the sensation of touching certain things. Some children will only wear one garment all the time. For some children touch may be painful, while others may seek restraint as they enjoy the sensation, seeking out 'pressure' touch and needing a firm hold for reassurance. Children may avoid having their hair and nails cut.

Hypo-sensitive – some children with autism have a low response to pain and may not report illness. They are at risk of burns or scalds. They may have self-injurious behaviour (such as nipping, pulling hair, scratching) but they are not setting out to injure or hurt themselves – they enjoy the sensation. They can become addicted to their own body's endorphins being released when they have pain and thus self-harm, for example pulling hair out because they like the sensation (trichotillomania).

Balance (vestibular)

Hyper-sensitive – an autistic child may have a fear of being moved (excitability, or excessive sensitivity of an organ or body part). They may panic if their feet are not on the ground and refuse to travel in vehicles. They have a preference for sitting or lying and some may show an avoidance of physical activity or have a marked reaction to movement, eg vomiting.

Hypo-sensitive – these autistic children may be sensation seekers, showing hyper-activity and restlessness. You may notice that many severely autistic children rock back and forth, hit themselves, or will twirl or swing and jump and stand on their tip toes. The child may enjoy sitting on a gym ball instead of a chair as they get the feeling of balancing.

Body position (proprioceptive)

Hyper-sensitive – some autistic children may have rigid body posture and movement and will turn their whole body around to look at something rather than just their head. Others may be fidgety and always moving around, unable to sit in one place. They may have difficulty with fine motor control and manipulation of objects eg, buttons.

Hypo-sensitive – some children may have poor body awareness and crash into things or fall over a lot, cannot negotiate doors very well, may tire easily and be noticed as being clumsy.

Other related factors (body temperature)

Hyper-sensitive – a child with autism may be very active, thirsty or distractible. They may strip off their clothes and prefer light clothing regardless of the weather conditions – this is because they are too hot (in addition to their sensory issues with touch).

Hypo-sensitive – they may feel the cold even when you think it is quite warm. They may insist on warm heavy clothing regardless of the weather.

Sensory processing (central auditory processing disorder)

Hyper-sensitive – an autistic child may have jumbled thoughts and be excitable, have poor concentration and be unable to process language unless it is written down. Others may interrupt and speak over people or they may have inattentiveness, hyper-activity and impulsiveness, which are characteristics of ADHD.

Hypo-sensitive – these children are slow to process information, getting stuck and having repetitive thoughts. If telling a story and interrupted the child may often have to start at the beginning again and retell the entire story. They may need prompts to be able to say what they are trying to tell you.

(www.autism.com/symptoms_sensory_overview and Shore 2004)

When you are visiting the home of a child with autism you should talk to the parents about the child's environment to ensure that these sensory difficulties are considered. See below for an example.

Scenario: Rebecca's room

Rebecca is eight years old and severely autistic. Rebecca's bedroom had posters on the wall of her favourite boy band, a mirror ball that shone bright lights of red, blue and white across the bedroom and a television. One wall also had striped wallpaper and she had all her toys on show with a clock on her bedside table. Rebecca could not settle to sleep, keeping her parents awake, and was always getting up, pacing around the room, pulling down the curtains and appearing to be over-stimulated. Her parents tried everything to settle Rebecca but they thought she was just disruptive. Rebecca's teacher noticed that she was tired at school and spoke to Rebecca's mother about this. Rebecca's mother was very upset that her behaviour was affecting her school day; Rebecca was falling asleep and her mother did not know how to manage this situation so she contacted the family centre for help.

A worker visited their home to discuss their referral. The support worker spoke to Rebecca's mother about how the bedroom was a likely contributory factor for some of Rebecca's behaviour. Rebecca's room was redecorated with plain beige walls, no posters and a plain blind on the window instead of a curtain. The television was removed, the mirror ball only used in the daytime, the clock was taken out of the room and her toys were kept in a cupboard when not in use. This meant that the environment was low arousal/stimulus and both Rebecca and parents slept well at night. Some of Rebecca's behaviour continued at other times but at night things were much better.

Rebecca's behaviour was her way of communicating that her environment was not working for her.

Activity: Wedding day

Samuel is a 10-year-old boy with severe autism, his mum Sue and father Michael have been invited to a close family member's traditional church wedding with a reception to follow, which includes a sit-down meal, and later on a disco with music and flashing lights. Sue and Michael have talked to you about their worries that Samuel has never been in a church before, let alone sat through a wedding. They have asked for support in helping to ensure that Samuel can attend the wedding without him going into crisis. This usually happens for Samuel if he enters a room full of people or other children: there have been difficulties getting him to school assemblies. Michael believes Samuel would be best in respite, but Erica does not feel it is fair that he misses out on special family occasions, and also points out that he would then not be in the wedding photos.

Considering the information shared in the communication chapter, perhaps you could help to draw an illustration that would help Samuel be prepared for what a wedding would involve, and also what the church looks like? What other things could you do to help prepare Samuel for the wedding, bearing in mind the sensory difficulties we have discussed above?

How can you include the reception and social dinner into the preparations for Samuel? Are there any other ways you could help his parents prepare Samuel for this event? Try and think of some solutions.

Methods and approaches for developing communication and learning

TEACCH approach

TEACCH (Treatment and Education of Autistic and Communication-Handicapped Children) has developed for both children and adults with autism. It focuses on the individual's skills, needs and interests and importantly is based on an understanding of the 'culture' of autism. It adapts to fit the individual's environment, building on their existing skills to increase their capacity to learn, comprehend and apply learning across different situations. It targets engagement, communication, social skills and executive functioning (mental skills that help the brain organise and act on information it receives to enable us to plan, remember things, prioritise, pay attention etc, and help us use information and experiences from the past to solve current problems). Strategies are targeted to the individual's ability and can be used by all those involved with the child, for example parents, other family, teachers and professionals in other settings, to ensure they are working together to deliver the different aspects of the programme.

TEACCH developed the intervention approach called 'Structured TEACCHing' as it fits with the structure that is based around the learning characteristics of those individuals with autism, and uses its environment, schedules and work systems, setting out clear and unambiguous expectations with visual materials to allow the person with autism (or ASD) to work as independently as possible within their different environments (such as school, home, in the community – on the bus or shops etc) and in different settings. TEACCH also draws on the strengths that many people with autism have, such as visual skills and good memory, which can help motivate them and build on their understanding of what they are doing (Mesibov 2004).

TEACCH uses the principles of cognitive behaviour therapy. The National Autistic Society offers a course on the TEACCH programme. Another approach that is very similar to TEACCH in its approach and complements TEACCH is SPELL.

SPELL

SPELL stands for Structure, Positive approaches and expectations, Empathy, Low arousal, Links. SPELL is used for both adults and children, building on their strengths and using evidence-based practice to support communication. Like many other approaches to support children with autism, SPELL uses the benefits of structure as this gives predictability and offers security and safety for the autistic child. Structure is believed to give autonomy and independence and allow the child to know what is happening around them. It uses Positive approaches and expectations to ensure that the person feels confident by developing the potential of the individual, following an assessment of their needs, which reinforces the individual's confidence as they develop their interests, strengths and abilities (as with TEACCH). This approach comes from the expectation that it is essential to see the world from the perspective of the child with autism, Empathise with how they experience their own world and what motivates them, understand their challenges and fears, and importantly respect them, thus helping develop their communication and reduce their anxiety. SPELL stresses the importance of the environment being one of Low arousal, ie calm with limited disruption, reducing stimuli that may affect their sensory processing difficulties. Finally, Links refers to the consistency offered from those closely involved with the child – parents, teachers and those in other familiar settings. They can provide a holistic approach to reduce inconsistencies and confusion by using the same strategies from their curriculum and other experiences in all aspects of the child's life (www.autism.org.uk). The National Autistic Society also offers courses in SPELL.

SCERTS

SCERTS is a comprehensive multi-disciplinary educational model for children with ASDs and their families. It supports their communication while helping prevent problem behaviour that affects a child's learning and ability to form relationships. SCERTS provides a framework for developing a comprehensive educational plan, based on core development challenges. It was designed to provide guidelines for helping children to become competent social communicators. SCERTS can be used to complement other approaches such as TEACCH, Social Stories or LEAP. The SCERTS model allows the child to achieve 'authentic progress', which is the ability to learn and spontaneously apply functional and relevant skills in a variety of settings with different people' (Prizant et al 2007).

SC – Social Communication: developing unprompted functional communication, emotional expression and secure and trusting relationships

ER – Emotional Regulation: developing the ability to sustain well-regulated emotions to cope with day-to-day situations and be available to learn and interact

TS – Transactional Support: developing support structures to respond to the child's needs and interests, help change and adapt the environment and offering strategies to support learning for those involved with the child.

The approach uses picture communication and schedules and sensory supports and includes individual evidence-based plans to enable education and emotional support for families and professionals in different settings (Prizant et al 2007). www.SCERTS.com. Autism Independent UK offers a training course for SCERTS: www.autismuk.com.

PECS

PECS stands for Picture Exchange Communication System and can be used for many children who have communication difficulties; however, PECS is particularly good for children with autism. As with TEACCH and SPELL it is visual and gives structure (using schedules) and routine to the child.

PECS works well for children with autism because it is simple and allows the child to request what they want. You may see PECS being used to tell a story, showing for example what is happening 'FIRST' and next 'THEN' (the wording can be different).

You need to tell Stephen that he has to do his work on his computer and then he is having his lunch. This may look like:

'FIRST'   **'THEN'**

Computer   Lunch

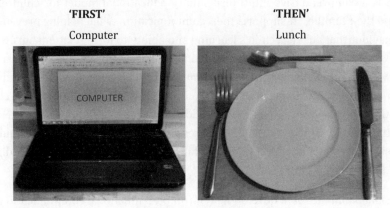

You can have a collection of familiar photographs or symbols that a child is able to choose and give to you to communicate what they want. You can use stick figures and drawings if you want to – anything that symbolises what is happening or what a child may want.

Children with autism can be rewarded when showing their skills in communicating, for example when they give you a PECS symbol showing a glass indicating they want a drink, you fill the glass with juice – they have their drink. Success! This is a 'concrete' reward. The rewards can be introduced slowly and then become more complex as the child becomes more effective at understanding how this method of communication works and its benefits. Once the child gets used to it they may often have a series of cues, showing a schedule of what is happening for them for example during a day. This child can understand the sequence over a longer period ie over the school day, but others may need the schedule breaking down even further.

schedule for an autistic boy

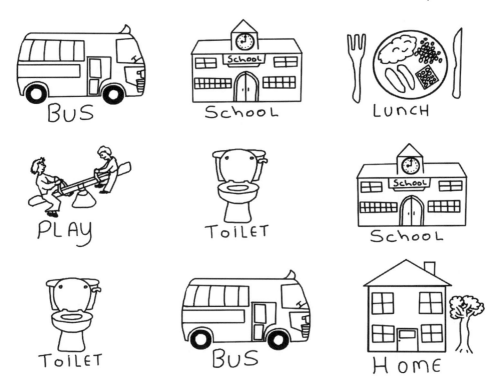

This schedule gives a short overview of what is happening for the child during the day. Children can be involved in making their schedule – often each picture is laminated with sticky velcro on the back, and they stick each one on a blank laminated sheet to build up their overall scenario. The child could for example take a picture of the toilet off the schedule and give this to the teacher to communicate that they need the toilet. This is only a very brief example of how it works and you can help parents use this type of communication with many different children with communication difficulties – they are no longer just used for children with autism. Many children may have their own photo album of their favourite and familiar symbols and photos that they use to communicate and these books can be replicated in all settings they use, for example school, home and respite care. Schools that cater for children with disabilities are very familiar with these methods of communication and can support parents implementing them at home.

You may have noticed that throughout this chapter there is a theme about schedules and how important they are for children and young people with varying disabilities, particularly those on the spectrum.

We know that we have only given you an overview of some of the difficulties and strategies for supporting communication and behaviour associated with autism, and as we said at the beginning of the chapter there is a great deal more that you can research about autism. We do hope, however, that this chapter has given you some things to consider to help you effectively work with children with autism.

Taking it further

Cohen, M J and Sloan, D L (2008) *Visual supports for people with autism: a guide for parents and professionals*. Bethesda, Maryland: Woodbine House.

Grandin, T (1995) *Thinking in pictures: And other reports from my life with autism*. New York: Doubleday.

McDonnell, A, McCreadie, M, Mills, R, Deyeau, R, Anker, R and Hayden, J (2015) The role of physiological arousal in the management of challenging behaviours in individuals with autistic spectrum disorders. *Research in Developmental Disabilities* Vol 35 January 2015 pp 311–322. Elsevier.

Savner, J L and Smith Myles, B (2000) *Making visual supports work in the home and community: strategies for individuals with autism and Asperger syndrome*. Shawnee Mission, Kansas: Autism Asperger Publishing Company.

You may want to give parents information about the Autism Helpline:

The National Autistic Society Your questions answered www.autism.org.uk/enquiry (accessed 2 January 2016).

Underside of the Iceberg Effect:

Region 15 Education Service Center The underside of the iceberg: Underlying characteristics of students on the autism spectrum www.netxv.net/cms/lib/TX07001386/Centricity/Domain/35/Handouts.pdf (accessed 10 January 2016).

This chapter focuses on how identifying needs around disabilities differs from general assessments, and how you will develop particular knowledge and skills from this field of social work. We talk you through using the Framework for the Assessment of Children in Need and their Families, while enabling you to fine tune your skills to identify the specific support needs. It will give an insight into the reality of practice that will enable you to consider some key points, situations and questions taken from real case scenarios.

Definition of disability

Statutory assessments under the Children Act 1989:

A child in need is defined under the Children Act 1989 as a child who is unlikely to achieve or maintain a satisfactory level of health or development, or their health and development will be significantly impaired, without the provision of services; or a child who is disabled... Children in need may be assessed under section 17 of the Children Act 1989, in relation to their special educational needs, disabilities, or as a carer... Under the Children Act 1989, local authorities are required to provide services for children in need for the purposes of safeguarding and promoting their welfare. Local Authorities undertake assessments of the needs of individual children to determine what services to provide and action to take. (Working Together to Safeguard Children 2015:17)

Regardless of their depth, all assessments should be linked to a plan that sets out what should happen to achieve the identified outcomes for the child or their family. We will talk about plans in further chapters, but for now we will focus on the assessment and analysis.

Multi-disciplinary working

Children with disabilities and/or complex health needs and their families are often in contact with a wide range of different agencies, and can be subject to multiple assessments.

The new 'Working Together to Safeguard Children 2015' guidance places an emphasis on the importance of early help in promoting the welfare of children, achieving positive outcomes and helping to achieve their full potential. These early help services are both critical for preventing the escalation into specialist services and an important 'step down' to those families who have been receiving a higher level of intervention.

In order to identify the most appropriate support an early assessment of the child's needs, an Early Help Assessment (EHA) will take place (formerly The Common Assessment Framework, CAF). The EHA is a standardised approach to assessing the needs of children and young people and considers the child's developmental needs, parental capacity and environmental factors. Through the delivery of the Early Help Offer, the use of EHA and the Team Around the Child (TAC) approach, once a difficulty is identified and assessed, help can be delivered by the most appropriate services and may be universal, targeted or specialist. If needs identified by the assessment cannot be met by a single agency or service, the response can be supported by agencies working together to support the family via a TAC model. The TAC brings together partner agencies and practitioners involved with the child/young person and their family. The TAC members will work together to identify the support necessary to deliver the needs from the EHA and appoint a Lead Professional (LP) to co-ordinate this support. The LP will be the key point of contact for the family and other professionals involved. Despite early intervention, some children and their families require more specialist help in order to achieve the identified outcomes. These families would usually progress to receiving services under the auspices of Child in Need s17 (if not deemed child protection s47). Consent is required from families to undertake an EHA (TAC and CIN s17) and to share information.

Boddy et al (2006:5) undertook research for the Department of Health around models of good practice in joined-up assessments when working for children with significant and complex needs, and noted how *'less attention has so far been paid to how to co-ordinate specialist assessments of children with more complex needs, for example assessments by social services, health services and special educational needs services.'* The research was commissioned as part of an ongoing Department for Education and Skills programme exploring the potential for joining up such multiple assessments for children with significant and complex health needs and/or disabilities. When working alongside other assessments it is worth considering the discourse around the social model versus the medical model. We suggest you explore this further but here we give a very brief overview. It is important to have an understanding of how these two models will affect the children and families you are working with, and it will also help you understand why when working with colleagues from a health background, they often have a different 'agenda' and see things differently, for example when undertaking a continuing care assessment (CCA) and exploring eligibility criteria.

Social model versus medical model

The social model of disability perspective is the principal model you will work with in your role as a social worker. It explores the person rather than the disability and will take into account environmental factors, including their home, and how a person with a disability is excluded from society in general because of their vulnerability and special needs. The social model aims to challenge discrimination and oppression and values individuals, eg if a person is a wheelchair user and requires access to a building but cannot do so because of steps, it is those steps that are viewed as the 'barrier', not the fact that the person uses a wheelchair.

The medical model focuses upon the illness or disability as the primary factor and views it as intrinsic to the individual. It will look at ways of managing the medical problems, eg by prescribing medication to manage a person's epilepsy. The medical model is essential for many children with complex health conditions and disabilities due to their multiple impairments, eg a person with cerebral palsy may have secondary conditions such as an inability to chew and swallow, breathing difficulties and problems with bladder or bowel control. They may also have some co-mitigating factors such as autism or asthma. You can see here why a person with such diagnoses would be heavily reliant on the medical model for their quality of life.

You may be allocated an assessment of need for a child with autism who has behavioural difficulties and a parent who is at their wits' end, stating they cannot cope and that there is a risk of family breakdown. During your assessment you would have to consider your recommendations: do you choose the social model, exploring behavioural strategies and cognitive behavioural therapies you can put in place to manage the behavioural difficulties, or do you consider the medical model with the view that the child should be prescribed medication to manage the behavioural outbursts and aggression linked to the autism? The latter may subdue the child and make him/her very sleepy and subdued, thus reducing or stopping the behavioural outbursts and allowing the parents to cope with the child and keep the family together; however, is it really addressing the causes of the behaviour or giving the parents strategies to manage their child? What would you do?

You may refer to CAMHS who would usually work with you and the child and family to look at the behavioural strategies first, with medication only being explored as a last resort.

You may be assessing a child who had a low birth weight, is not taking their feed and not meeting their milestones. You need to consider whether this is failure to thrive

(FTT) and, if so, is it organic or non-organic? For example, is it neglect (non-organic) due to actions of the caregiver or due to a medical or genetic reason (organic) such as the child having a condition like cystic fibrosis or cerebral palsy that makes it more difficult for the body to absorb nutrition. When assessing FTT it is important to be open-minded and consider both organic and non-organic factors, including unintentional factors such as a mother's inability to breastfeed, and those associated with neglect, eg poor attachment (Block et al 2005). The term FTT has become more recently known as faltering growth.

When working with children with disabilities, or who may have an undiagnosed disability, this can be a very complex assessment and multi-agency joint working with health colleagues is essential, using social and medical models in tandem. Health visitors will be key, helping give advice and support, and may contact you with any worries they have that a child is not reaching their milestones, particularly when associated with non-organic concerns – for example if they are worried about neglect and parental capacity to meet the child's needs. Many children may already have diagnosed conditions that could be linked to FTT. Boys and girls have different percentile charts, with boys tending to be bigger than girls, and consideration may need to be given to children from different racial and cultural backgrounds and to the parents' features and characteristics, ie if the parents are tall or short. Obesity is more often acquired although there may be hereditary factors to consider.

As you enter into the specialist role of assessing a family caring for a child with a disability and or complex health needs, you will be introduced to a range of new terminologies, conditions, diagnoses, prescriptive and medical models and interventions. Within this multi-disciplinary set of professionals you will need to communicate, liaise, co-ordinate and facilitate meetings, and you will often take the lead role in all of this. For example, a child may have a heart condition overseen by a specialist at Leicester Royal Infirmary, and epilepsy that is managed by a neurologist in Sheffield. They may also have their local paediatrician, child development centre, community paediatric nurses, support care staff, early help professionals, specialist educational professionals, physio and occupational therapists, speech and language and orthotics involved. These are just a few of the main players involved and there are many children who have all of these and more at any given time.

There may be cases that require your involvement in discharge planning meetings, where you will contribute to ensuring that there is a clear support plan for the family when their child is allowed home. Best practice sees an assessment being allocated at the earliest point, for example when a young baby is on the neonatal ward, and where discharge planning goes hand in hand with the assessment of need and identification of support needs.

Scenario: Paul

Paul is a young baby born prematurely with complicated breathing problems and a heart condition. Paul needs 24-hour oxygen and is about to be discharged from the neonatal ward. An assessment of need has been requested by the charge nurse on the ward to look at support needs for Paul when he is at home with his parents.

Points to consider: as Paul requires 24-hour oxygen it may be that he would meet the criteria for continuing healthcare. This is a bit like an extension of hospital care at home, with support from nursing care to maintain the level of healthcare needed. It is useful to understand how the CCA works and informs decisions around health funding and support for a family, and this may relate to the social care elements of your assessment. CCAs are explained further in this chapter when looking at assessing in reality, but for now, just to get your thought processes flowing, have a go at considering the few questions contained in the activity below. (We discuss Continuing Care in more detail in Chapter 9.)

Activity

Thinking about multi-disciplinary working, what do you think needs to happen before Paul is discharged home?

How best can you pull the information together from all the relevant health professionals to complete your assessment in such a short time?

What are the challenges or complicating factors that you may be faced with?

Which people and professionals do you need to invite to the meeting?

While the health service will be focusing on the child's health and medical needs from a clinical approach, you need to consider the child and their family's social care needs, and this is where your assessment will be important in identifying the appropriate levels of support. Your assessment may identify the need for further specialist assessments, which would define the more specific needs of the child, for example CAMHS, speech and language, occupational therapy or psychological assessments. It is important that these other assessments are co-coordinated so that the child does not become lost between the different agencies involved and their different procedures. Having an awareness of the various professional disciplines, with their respective roles and responsibilities, will be beneficial to you in informing your assessments. The different professionals you will meet, as well as family members and carers involved with the child, will enable you to draw from their different perspectives, giving you a more complete picture of the child and their world.

A holistic assessment should consider:

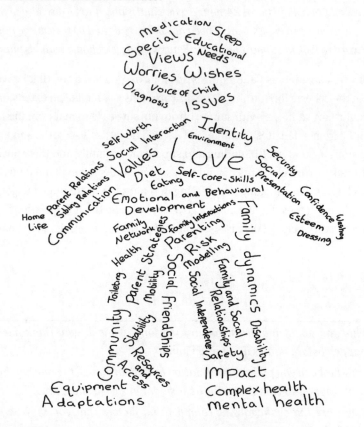

Taking time to research and plan

Being introduced to illnesses, syndromes, diagnoses and health conditions that are new to you can seem daunting at first. Unfortunately, there are no short cuts through this as you can only develop through experience, research and talking to the people with specialist knowledge. Try to not rush in without taking some time to prepare, plan and organise yourself. As with most new allocated social care cases, the first step to take is to read the case file and chronologies. With consent speak to people in the know, such as paediatric nurses or other health staff, to find out about specific conditions and how they affect the individual child.

Remember that with each child's assessment there will be other contributing factors that make the child's situation unique to them. For example, as well as their disability there may be complicating factors around their family environment.

There are ecological theoretical models to help map the needs. The assessment framework is derived from Bronfenbrenner's theory of ecological systems. They each look at other contributing factors around a child, including their family and their environments, which make each child's experience of life and their specific condition unique.

Much of contemporary developmental psychology is the science of the strange behavior of children in strange situations with strange adults for the briefest possible periods of time. (Bronfenbrenner, 1977: 513)

Use appropriate medical information sites to learn about illnesses, as this helps to understand their impact and how the child's development may be impaired or affected. Be aware not to use 'unofficial' websites and only put information into your assessments that is factual and correct. Developing this knowledge helps you to communicate and discuss needs with the family, and it is possible sometimes to find information that parents did not know which can be helpful to them. Having some knowledge also helps to give parents and carers more confidence in your abilities to assess and support them. Please understand that you are *not* expected to become an expert in health matters and it is important that you do not give the impression that you are an expert in the field because you have done some research. A little bit of knowledge is enough, and if parents or carers ask advice around medical matters you can direct them to the appropriate professional. You are demonstrating that you have awareness and understanding only.

Drawing from parents' expertise and experience

Parents and carers will usually have in-depth knowledge of their child's condition and so will be able to explain it to you. Remember they are living the larger and fuller version of the snapshot you will get on your visits. They will tell you how it is for them and you will also be able to observe their experience in parts. There will be some parents who are desperate to receive support or respite and will describe their worst days and their most difficult experiences, while other parents may be embarrassed about their child's behaviour and try to minimise their real needs, feeling that they are being a nuisance asking for help despite a genuine need. Active listening will help you hear what is not being said.

You will need to be mindful of the pain that some parents undergo when having to repeatedly describe the symptoms and conditions of their child, and judge this when they are sharing their information. Furthermore, some parents may be finding it difficult to talk about or even accept their situation (see Chapter 3). Your information gathering will be crucial in these circumstances, and needs to capture a true reflection of the child and their family's support needs.

Some parents may be taking their child home for the first time, so they are facing new territory themselves as well as coping with the significant changes that taking a child with disabilities home will bring to their life. As a social worker and assessor you will be able to share parts of this journey with them, supporting them through this process and enabling them to identify and cope with the effects of their situation.

Parents with a learning disability

There are many reasons why a child may have a disability, such as a prenatal infection, traumatic birth and being starved of oxygen, brain injury at birth or brain damage after their birth, perhaps a result of an accident. When a child has a disability, you should consider if there are any genetic causal factors, which may also indicate that one or more of the child's parents have a learning disability, not ruling out that a parent with a learning disability may have a child that does not have any learning or physical disabilities. The Working Together to Safeguard Children (2010) document *'estimates that there are 985,000 people in England with a learning disability... and estimates of the number of adults with learning disabilities who are parents vary widely from 23,000 to 250,000.'* (DCSF 2010:279)

When you are undertaking an assessment of need for a child whose parent has a learning disability do not make generalisations and assumptions. Even though one or more parents may have a learning disability, this does not mean that they are neglectful parents. When parents are not supported appropriately and early intervention is not put in place, however, their children may suffer neglect due to omission (DCSF 2010:279). You must ensure that parents understand why an assessment is being completed, what is being asked of them, that the information is in a form that is accessible to them and they understand what they are giving consent to. Brandon et al (2009), who studied serious case reviews, found in 15% of cases parents had a learning disability. It is good practice to work with colleagues from Adult Social Care where necessary; depending on their level of disability they may not meet criteria for a service but should be entitled to an assessment in their own right to determine this. If a parent with learning difficulties is not deemed as being eligible for a service from Adult Social Care, services may have to be put in place by Children's Services to support their parenting needs if this is deemed necessary to avoid the child being at risk of harm.

Parents with learning disabilities may know what they need to do to meet the basic care needs for their child, ie giving food, drink and shelter, but they may require help with putting appropriate routines in place, and as the child grows up, putting boundaries in place and ensuring the child is stimulated. They may not consider dangers within the home and both environmental factors and parental capacity should be given more consideration when a parent has a disability. The impact of a parent's disability may become more profound as the child reaches their middle childhood. Parents with disabilities may not be able to support the child's learning due to their own lack of understanding; for example, the parent may have difficulty reading and writing and thus be unable to support their child with homework, or the parent's own experiences in school may colour the child's attendance and how this is prioritised. Their child may have behavioural difficulties due to the lack of boundaries during their earlier childhood. The child may also become a carer to their parents. Good support networks are essential and this could come through relatives or grandparents or other universal and targeted services (DH 2007).

Regardless of the type of assessment you are undertaking, be it s17 Child in Need, s47 to establish significant harm or an early help assessment, all needs relating to the parent's learning disability should be considered alongside the child's individual needs. You should give further consideration to a parent with a disability (including sensory disabilities) who is parenting a child with a disability, particularly if the child's disability is severe and profound. For example, the child may have complex feeding regimes or require suction or ventilation. You need to work with health colleagues to assess if parents are able to meet the needs of their child's disability in addition to their basic care needs, and ensure appropriate training is provided and regular reviews are undertaken where necessary.

Fabricated or induced illnesses

It is important that you clarify and confirm self-reported illnesses or conditions with the appropriate health professionals, or ask to see clinical and health reports that give a definite description and confirmation of diagnosis and prescribed medications. Safe practice is around not recording information as fact on the assessment when it is reported and only given by the parent or carer. It is important to remember that once information is written into your assessment it will be taken by others as fact and may be read by other professionals to inform future assessments or even shared in court, therefore clarity about diagnoses and conditions is essential.

You need to be very clear in the assessment about whether information has been shared by parents, for example your report would state 'Mum informed that Jonny has a diagnosis of epilepsy.' To firm up your reporting, this should be followed up and confirmed by the health professional so that it would say 'Jonny was diagnosed with epilepsy in 2003 when he was two years old by Dr Bubble, consultant neurologist.' In most cases parents will innocently mistake a consultant's suggestions or exploration of a condition for a diagnosis, and there may be further tests and assessments to confirm the diagnosis or condition. This needs clarifying and can be reported as pending further tests and confirmation. Parents are often desperate for answers and for their child to be given a diagnosis. (See Chapter 2 for more information.)

Assessing in reality

Think about the assessment framework and what the key areas are. How are you going to gather the information from parents? There are various theories to help you approach this, such as the questioning model, the exchange model, the appreciative model and many others. No matter which approach or eclectic mix of approaches you decide to use, it is usually best to explain to the family how you will need to make notes to ensure that you keep the information they share as accurate as possible. Some parents will wait for questions to be asked while others may want to just tell you their story – the latter promotes the opportunity for active listening and adept note taking to pick up key issues from their narrative. Try to imagine how it feels to be in their shoes, having someone taking down what you say, and how hard this can be for people, especially in the presence of a social worker. Never be afraid to be honest and explain how you understand how difficult this may be for them, and let them know how you are trying to make them feel at ease during your visit. It is a great skill that you will develop to be able to be actively listening, observing, interacting and taking notes without the family seeing you just scribbling all the time. Stepping into their shoes is an element of the appreciative model, where the questioning can be an enabling technique for parents to develop an appreciation of how life is for their child. Very often parents will want and need to tell you the difficulties from their perspective as carers, which is part and parcel of assessing the impact on them in caring for the child's complex needs. In order to keep the child and their own needs in focus, however, it is good practice to remind and guide parents and carers of this concept too. You will be able to explore this further in the activity that concludes this chapter.

The simplistic way of explaining an assessment to families is to say that it is your role to draw a clear picture of the child and their family that represents and identifies their needs. This has been explained before in terms of decision makers at resource panels who have not met or seen the family and yet have to make decisions that affect the child's life. It is best explained that a detailed and clear assessment helps the decision makers imagine how it is for the child and their family. This, as always, should include positives and things that are working well (Signs of Safety model) as well as difficult issues for the family and what they are worried about.

It is likely that you will be working within a team that has Signs of Safety (SOS) embedded within their practice. The SOS model is a risk assessment and case planning format that is meaningful for professionals as well as the parents and children. It turns social care practice and intervention on its head, takes away the jargon, and gives families the opportunity to take control of their own plans for change by drawing from their own family support networks. It is also clear about what agencies are worried about and what they need to do as a family in order to take these worries away. Currently almost 200 agencies in 13 countries, including Australia, New Zealand, Japan, Canada, the USA and across Europe, including the UK, are implementing the SOS model, pioneered in Australia by Steve Edwards and Dr Andrew Turnell in the late 1990s. Although primarily a model used in child protection based on danger statements, safety goals and plans, SOS can be adapted to fit in all aspects of practice and is a particularly useful tool to inform assessments, identify next steps and outcomes, for recommendations and to inform future planning. Using the model you will 'map' cases, exploring complicating factors and barriers through the questioning framework that helps keep a focus on the key issues to be addressed and to prevent drift. Some people use danger statements and safety goals in their analysis, which allows for clear and descriptive language to present a clear picture of the child's world, the worries and the minimum expectations upon families that would allow the case to be closed (Turnell and Murphy 2014).

The Framework for the Assessment of Children in Need and their Families

Many assessments undertaken in social care are completed using the Framework for the Assessment of Children in Need and their Families (DH 2000), which uses a holistic and ecological approach to exploring the child's needs, with them as the central focus of all contributing factors.

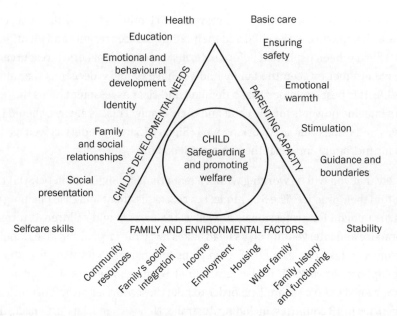

Figure 6.1 Assessment triangle. 'Moving on from bowlby: theories about child development' https://movingonfrombowlby.wordpress.com/tag/assessment-framework/ (accessed 21 August 2015)

Continuing care assessments

A child with a disability can present with a whole range of differing and complex health conditions and behaviours that can affect their daily living and impair their development and learning. Some children present with such complex health issues, perhaps a life-limiting condition, that they may require a specific assessment of their continuing healthcare; these use the National Framework for Children and Young People's Continuing Care (DH 2010c) to determine the level of continued healthcare that needs to be provided to keep the child at home with sufficient support and care in place. '*A continuing care package will be required when a child or young person has needs arising from disability, accident or illness that cannot be met by existing universal or specialist services alone*' (DH 2010c:10). This assessment would often be carried out in parallel to your own and be completed by a health professional, eg community paediatric nurse or school nurse.

Parents of children with complex health needs may find themselves having to be trained to carry out procedures on their child that are of a nursing nature. For example, when a child has a percutaneous endoscopic gastrostomy (PEG) tube fitted in the stomach it needs cleaning and constant care, as well as the parent having to cope with not being able to bottle or spoon feed their child. A tracheotomy tube needs to be suctioned to clean out the mucus and keep the tube clear to ensure oxygen gets through and the child can breathe. The tube goes through the child's neck, so the wound needs to be kept clean and sterile and the whole tracheotomy tube has to be changed on a regular basis: parents and family members will have to undertake training in order to continue this care at home. The effects can show in many different ways, with one mother describing how she felt more like her child's nurse than a mum and that this was affecting her bonding with the child.

Impact on parent/carers

As an assessor working closely with the family you will observe a range of parenting styles, values, cultures and beliefs. You will already understand how parenting in general brings many responsibilities and challenges with regard to meeting children's basic needs. You will also discover how for many parents, parenting in general is not always easy. Moreover, when a parent has a child with a disability, they are faced with significant changes to their lives. The reality of the care, commitment and supervision required is above and beyond everyday expectations, often leaving parents physically exhausted and emotionally drained. The key component of an assessment is to explore this impact on parents and family members in their roles of looking after and living with a child with a disability, while keeping the child and their needs as the central focus.

Disability Living Allowance applications are considered by measuring the care elements that are required for a child above and beyond what would be required for any child on a day-to-day basis. It is a similar concept that helps you to identify the extra care that parents have to provide and the stresses and strains this places upon them as carers.

In some families, there are other contributing factors that make their caring role even more difficult and can create barriers and complications; for example, parents may have illness or mental health issues, or may be isolated from a supportive family network.

Activity: **So what is the difference when assessing disabilities?**

Taking one of the domains of the 'Assessment Triangle' (shown on p 144), let's take a different perspective. Here we consider the impact of disabilities and imagine how these difficulties would look to an observer of a family. We have helped you by starting this activity using examples of children with a severe level of autism. See if you can finish it by filling in the gaps before doing one on your own.

Parenting capacity	**Basic care**
Area of need	*Some children and young people are fully reliant on others to provide their basic needs; some reach adulthood and continue with this need.*
How would this affect a family?	Ongoing use of nappies long after a child may have been toilet trained.
	Moving and handling may be difficult due to the size of the young person or their physical disability.
	Feeding may need to continue at regular intervals, even through the night.
	Parents and carers are continuing to provide a high level of care above and beyond age and milestone expectations.
	Sleep may not be established as a routine, which would allow rest and recharge for parents.
What would this look like?	Tired and exhausted parents.
	Family routines in disarray.
	High levels of stress and tension within family relationships.
	Ensuring safety
Area of need	*Some children may have no awareness of dangers, road safety or hazards. Some may require one-to-one supervision at all times and some may require a higher ratio of adult/carer support around the home and out in the community.*
How would this affect a family?	

What would this look like?	
Emotional warmth	
Area of need	*Some children will have difficulty understanding their own feelings and the feelings of others. This can be difficult for parents who in showing their love and affection find it is not reciprocated.*
How would this affect a family?	
What would this look like?	Grief and loss for parents and other members of the family. There may be a lack of understanding where parents view behaviour as naughty or rude.
Stimulation	
Area of need	*Some children may have a high need for sensory feedback that meets their own range of needs, such as spinning, smelling, tasting, repeated movements, counting, stroking, feeling, visual and vestibular movements.*
How would this affect a family?	
What would this look like?	Grief and loss. The child may have significant and global development delay, making it difficult for them to learn to read, write and communicate.
Guidance and boundaries	
Area of need	*A child with autism will often have added needs around their learning and cognitive development, and may have difficulty in understanding and following rules and expectations placed upon them. They will often follow their own agenda and parents may be finding it difficult to engage them in family routines and structures.*
How would this affect a family?	
What would this look like?	

It is easy sometimes to fall into the role of the 'fixer' and want to put support and interventions in place to help with situations; however, families mostly want to be able to find their own solutions, without social care intervention. The danger of being a fixer is creating a dependency culture. The skilled assessor will look at strengths, wealth and family support networks before looking to source provisions, resources and services. For example, Ben may have grandparents who will care for him overnight on a regular basis, which provides much needed respite for his mum. This respite may be enough to meet her needs, rather than having to put in external resources. You should always consider this first and use universal support in the first instance.

Sibling focus

When assessing impact, it is important to include siblings of the child with a disability, as very often with the child requiring so much care and attention, the siblings may have become young carers, trying to support their parents, or more often, especially when the child with a disability is presenting with challenging behaviour, the sibling may be retreating to their bedroom for solace and escape, which can lead to a cycle of invisibility or isolation. A younger brother of 14 years old spoke of never having been able to spend quality time alone with his parents before, but he loved his brother and understood his needs. You may find in your assessments that you identify that the siblings are taking on a caring role, either helping to care for the child with a disability directly or for their parents, for example helping to prepare meals, shop, clean, do laundry and other roles around the home. You might see some siblings having to miss out on social opportunities because it is difficult for them to go out or invite friends round for sleepovers, parties etc. Some children may be caring for a parent with a disability or illness, or substance abuse issues, while also caring for their sibling with a disability. All these young people are recognised as young carers and their world is important to include in your assessment; your analysis will take into account how their lives are being affected and how they could access support for themselves. Young Carers Groups are talked about in Chapter 3.

Points for further consideration prior to assessment

The first and most important step is to discuss the assessment with your supervisor/manager, get clarity as to what is expected from your involvement and what the key issues are. You need to try and determine if there are any known risks you need to be aware of: your safety comes first and foremost. While your manager has a duty of care, you also have a responsibility for your own safety, so don't be afraid to check out risks, especially in terms of assessing young people displaying aggressive outbursts and challenging behaviour.

In practice we are advised not to be reactive, as this can often lead to poor decision making and irrational interventions that do not support the needs presented, so be mindful of just jumping in and muddling through the assessment, as this can make you appear unprofessional and disorganised. Aspire to produce quality assessments as these will form the foundations of your professional acknowledgement and development. There will be many critics who will be quick to highlight your errors, so give yourself time for reading and planning and let the family meet their organised, prepared and informed social worker, as this will inspire their confidence and trust in you.

Each case should have a chronology. Read the chronology if an up-to-date one is available; our experience has taught us that sometimes in a very busy and stressed team they may not be completed or up to date. Good practice is to start a chronology upon your allocation and then try to update it as you go along. This will help give a flavour of the issues presented and to highlight any patterns in behaviours or situations that have occurred.

Take note of involved people and professionals, old and current. These will be valuable in ascertaining background information to inform your assessment. It is important during the initial visits to complete a 'genogram' with the family. This will help build a picture of their support networks and consider the available family resources and wealth.

These people can then be involved in completing a support plan or emergency plan; for example if a parent is hospitalised the plan can be put in place so that the child with a disability is cared for by familiar people who know them well. This is particularly important for children who have complex health needs and may need a trained network of carers, eg who could be called upon in an emergency to help with a child who needs a gastrostomy feed.

Remember you will need consent first before contacting professionals; it's just good at this point to list any relevant people and their contact details so they are ready.

The diagram below shows an example of a genogram.

An example of a genogram

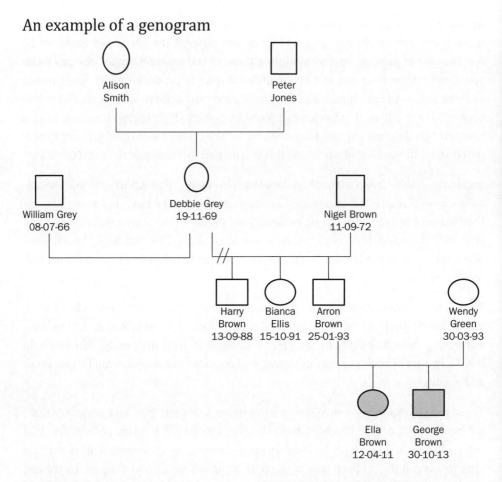

Reading is also essential to understanding what has gone on and which interventions have already been put in place. There is nothing worse than suggesting a service or a strategy to a family only for them to tell you 'I have done that and it did not work' early on in the relationship: it can start you off on a negative footing as the family feel that they've been here before and are going round in circles. You need to give the impression that you are a fresh person who can bring new ideas to the table. You need to read what has been delivered before. You may feel that there is something they did not try for long and want to suggest they give it another go; you need to be prepared with an explanation for why they should revisit this strategy, so you need to explore who did the work and what the barriers were. Parents do respond to praise themselves, though some will panic as they will not be used to hearing it and will also worry that they will not get the support they need if everything is looking a lot better; in these cases you can talk with them about what remaining barriers or complicating factors there are to their success (SOS). When a family have had long-term social work involvement they may feel low and inadequate as they will have had many years of being told where they are going wrong. With you as their new social worker, hearing any positive observations will help to build your working relationship with them.

If there is a transfer of social worker or other agencies, for your first contact there should be a joint visit arranged so the preceding worker can visit and make introductions with you. Ensure you update all addresses and telephone numbers on file. Be aware that some families will be unhappy about changes in social workers as they may have had many different social workers involved with their child, even though these changes may have been unavoidable.

If you are making the visit alone from a referral, make sure that you have spoken with the referrer first to check that they have informed the parents about your involvement. This is also a good opportunity to check out the outcomes required by the referrer in relation to why they have requested your involvement. This should marry up with what your supervisor has told you: you need to be careful of professionals adding roles that have not been put on the referral and which may not be in your remit. This has sometimes happened during an introductory visit to a family's home and roles have been explained to them that have not been previously agreed. This is a difficult situation for the social worker, and why contact with the referrer is important to clarify their expectations before any visit is made.

There are many different reasons for assessment, from parents requesting support for their child with a disability, a safeguarding assessment, or a concern that has been shared by a member of the public or another agency. If the assessment is in relation to safeguarding, you need to be closely guided by your supervisor as you progress and find further information, as it may be necessary for the assessment to progress to a Child Protection Procedure under Section 47. This is where you will need to consult the guide to inter-agency working to safeguard and promote the welfare of children, 'Working Together to Safeguard Children' (DfE 2015).

Talk with your supervisor about what they expect from the assessment in terms of their initial hypothesis. Your supervisor may have background information about the family from previous involvement, or it may be that services are already in place and the family has requested additional support. Finally, ensure that you use your supervision appropriately and discuss your assessment with your manager as you progress through it.

Developing your analysis

Once you have gathered all the information you will need to make decisions and recommendations based on your findings from the assessment. You will need to consider the family's own strengths and wealth in terms of their parenting attributes, resilience and how they are supported within their network of family and friends.

Your analysis should be a summary of the child and their world, looking at their basic social, emotional, communication, health, educational, care, cultural and religious needs. Try to think about how their world is for them. Are they safe, healthy, developing as well as they could be? Are they surrounded by people who love and care for them? Are they getting to their health appointments? Are they attending school? You will also be considering the information you have gathered around the surrounding and environmental factors, such as housing, home conditions, family dynamics, isolation etc. Within each of these areas you will have gained an overview of how and if these needs are met, partly met or unmet. To develop your analysis you might want to question your thoughts and hypothesise around the unmet needs. What are the barriers? What is getting in the way of the family meeting these needs? What are the complicating factors making it difficult for the parents? Why are they finding it so difficult? How can they manage or continue as they are? Use the SOS model, asking what are we worried about? What's working well? What needs to happen?

Social care involvement is not always about intervention or services that are put in place to meet the unmet need. Some families will want the social worker to step in to put things in place for them perhaps when it is not really needed or because they are just too tired or stressed. Some will want respite services because a friend has it for their child. Some families will just need you to inform them of community activities and support they can access universally without further social care involvement. There will be some families who will be trying their best to manage and are not expecting services despite there being a clear need for support. Remember you need to focus on *need* and not *want*.

By exploring the barriers and complicating factors you may identify what needs to happen to reduce or remove the barriers. You will be deciding whether you think that the family are well equipped with their own support wealth and resources, or if they need support, what kind of support and at what level. A good analysis demonstrates a balance of strengths around supporting the child, with a clear description of the contributing factors around any unmet needs, and have some well thought out, viable suggestions and recommendations for positive outcomes for the child. There is a fine balance in getting this right and each child you assess will be unique and individual and will strengthen your analytical skills and experience. Remember your analysis is not a 'cut and paste' of the information from your assessment but neither should you be introducing anything new into your analysis. It needs to be where you make your argument using your supporting evidence by differentiating the views and reasons for why you have chosen your desired outcome.

To conclude, you remind the reader of how you proved your argument, keeping it brief and succinct, then you can give your final recommendation, eg that Jonny has a short break or receives services to meet his personal care needs.

You will find it an investment to develop a wide knowledge base about the services and activities that are available for families in the area you are working within. There are universal services available to children with disabilities who provide activities at little or no cost, and which can also provide some short respite breaks for parents. See Chapter 9 when considering help for families.

Taking it further

Early Help Assessments: each local authority will have their own Local Offer – search online for EHA and your local authority for more details.

Further guidance can be accessed at:

H M Government (2009) Safeguarding Disabled Children – Practice Guidance. Available online www.gov.uk/government/uploads/system/uploads/attachment_data/file/190544/ 00374-2009DOM-EN.pdf (accessed 22 March 2015).

H M Government (2010) Recognised, valued and supported: Next steps for the Carers Strategy. Available online www.gov.uk/government/uploads/system/uploads/attachment_data/ file/213804/dh_122393.pdf (accessed 22 March 2015).

Department of Health (2010b) *National Framework for Children and Young People's Continuing Care*. DH London www.dh.gov.uk

Murray, M and Osborne C and The Children's Society (2009) *Safeguarding Disabled Children: Practice Guidance*. The Children's Society: DCSF Publications: Nottingham You can download copies of this document at www.teachernet.gov.uk/publications.

Chapter 7 | Exploring behaviour management techniques and strategies

This chapter will give a flavour of the challenges parents face when living with a child with a disability and their related behaviours. It will enable you to explore different strategies around managing behavioural difficulties, linking in with Chapter 4. It will discuss some of the challenges for parents in terms of balancing the general concept of behaviour with risk management and safety planning. We explore how a child can be defined by their behaviour and how this behaviour can affect the whole family. It will enable you to consider some of the training strength-based programmes used, which enable parents to develop and improve their approaches to managing their child's behaviour. This chapter will share examples of how CAMHS can support you and be a key partner agency when working with children with disabilities.

For a parent to fully understand their child's disability-related behaviour is as difficult as a brand new parent learning to understand their new role and responsibilities.

Parents of children with disabilities are faced with daily dilemmas of trying to balance their rules and boundaries in keeping with their child's disability; they may have difficulty in recognising the need to adapt their general concepts of behavioural expectations. Some parents will have over-compensated and made allowances for their child, which has then presented them with challenges and patterns of behaviour that are hard to undo once established and learned as acceptable. An example is that parents often allow their child to sleep in their bedroom because they are difficult to settle at night, getting the child used to the parent being there and then behavioural outbursts when they try to put the child in their own room. The parent gives in and allows the child to stay in their bedroom (sometimes even in their bed). This becomes habitual and very difficult to break, with the parents wanting to settle for 'a quiet life'. The authors have experienced parents still having a child in their bedroom into their teenage years. There may be difficulties for parents faced with the need to balance house rules among siblings who are expected to follow a different set of rules. This can often leave a child feeling badly done to or developing resentment towards their sibling as they feel that it is unfair for them to have to comply with a more rigid set of rules. This may cause conflict in relationships and disrupt harmony within the family. In some cases it can result in families becoming dysfunctional and close to breaking down completely.

Key factors that contribute to behaviours

There are three main factors to understand and consider when working with and supporting children with disabilities and their families.

Parents' understanding: Parents' understanding of their child's disability, what the disability means to them and what they understand of the impact the disability may have on their child's learning and understanding. Parents may have unrealistic expectations of their child and how they will manage their child's behaviours when they are unable to meet these expectations. Conversations with parents to explore these issues will help you understand their expectations and the barriers they come across in trying to get their child to be able to respond and comply.

The child's understanding: The child's level of understanding and their thought processing ability levels, in other words how much they can understand their own behaviours, consequences and problem solving, and the expectations placed upon them by the rules and boundaries in their everyday life. Get to know the child and their disability to ascertain:

» their level of understanding – you need to explore their thought processes

» their cognitive levels of understanding

» how they communicate and express their wishes and feelings

» how they identify with themselves and their disability

» their strengths and their barriers, eg to communication, mobility, sensory impairment

» their understanding of the behaviours they present

» if they are aware and able to plan, or if they are reactive to situations and unable to problem solve or see the consequences of their actions?

It is also important to explore the communication between family members and the child and how effective or ineffective this may be.

The environment: Looking at the environment in which the child lives is important to consider, as there may be factors that are causing barriers and difficulties for the child and their family. For example, a child may be living in a very small house and has a physical disability and therefore he is lifted and carried around the house. Occupational therapy have not been able to make appropriate adaptations for various reasons, such as the house is too small for mobile equipment or it is rented from a private landlord who does not allow any adaptations to be made. It may be that the child is not sleeping and shares a bedroom with a sibling who is kept awake at night and thus struggling at school due to lack of sleep.

The home and bedroom for the child may be cluttered and this may be creating information and sensory overload, which could be a major factor in the behaviours that are presented by the child. Parents who are not aware of the need to keep their child's bedroom a low arousal environment (clear and plain), in order to provide a calming place for their child to settle and sleep, may be thinking that their child needs all their toys available to them. Research has shown that children who are deprived of sleep are more prone to present with challenging behaviours during the day. The Sleep Clinic, a registered charity, gives support and advice to parents about sleep routines. Sleep practitioners will help them put together a sleep plan and continue to support parents while they implement the plan (see 'Taking it further' at the end of the chapter).

The home environment, in particular the routines and care patterns that are established by parents as ways of meeting their child's needs and the learned responses that develop, can also create specific associations for children with learning-related disabilities. Parents may find it difficult to understand why their child behaves completely differently at home than they do in other settings, which can create a sense of failure or disappointment in parents who see others succeed in helping a child to take next steps when they are struggling to move their child on.

Using resources that are around the child and their family is valuable in terms of enabling change and progress. Parents can find themselves stuck in a situation, and this is where being a social worker enables you to observe them with an objective eye and then build and develop ways to support and enable the family to develop solutions, and also to recognise the resources and ideas that are around them.

Pitching it at the right level

Some parents may get stressed, frustrated or angry with their child when they do not respond or comply with their expectations. This is especially seen when a child has low cognitive development for their age. It can become difficult for a child who does not understand the concept of consequences and discipline, such as 'being grounded', sent up to their room or made to do chores. Furthermore, there may be parents who feel the need to carry over discipline for previous misdemeanours, for example 'You're not going on your iPad because of your behaviour yesterday.' To a child with a brain injury, development disorder or global development delay, it can be difficult to recall previous events as their functioning level is running from moment to moment, mostly in the now, thus they do not understand why they are being punished.

In your supporting role you may need to identify the child's actual levels of cognitive learning and understanding, and perhaps have these explained by the professionals who have monitored and measured them. If this is shown in a school report, it can be difficult for parents to translate what they mean for their child, especially if schools talk about eg P levels, which is a common term in specialist educational settings. If it is a report by an educational psychologist, there will be charts and scales and complex language used. (P levels are a set of levels that sit before the curriculum academic levels, mostly used to enable children with special educational needs to still have levels of achievement, aimed at their level of development and pace.) It would be invaluable to the family if you could get these reports summarised to show a comparison with age-equivalent levels the child is functioning at. This in itself can help reduce the child's difficult behaviours which can stem from frustration borne out of overly high parental expectations.

Case study: Joe

Joe is a ten-year-old boy. His parents, George and Mary, have complained to his social worker, Francine, that when they give him several instructions he often forgets what he has been asked to do. Francine reviews the summary of the educational psychologist's report, which shows him functioning at a four-year-old stage of development and understanding. She explains the report to George and Mary. As they understand its implications they begin to lower their expectations and see more success in Joe's behaviour. They give him instructions one at a time and at his own level and so his understanding grows. Whereas before Mary would have said to Joe, 'Go upstairs, brush your teeth and get your coat as we are going soon', she now understands that he cannot take on so much information and is overloaded. By the time she had finished giving such a long instruction, Joe had forgotten what was said and perhaps had reached the stairs and thought – now what? Too much information all at once with too great an expectation may have resulted in Mary thinking Joe was being insolent and ignoring her, thus getting him into trouble and beginning to act out behaviours.

Extended family members will need to adjust and develop an understanding of the disability related behaviours and needs in order that they can support the family. It may be that a child is born profoundly deaf and his parents may need to learn new communication methods: other members of the family would need to learn these too so that communication is effective in the whole family.

Adapting the general behaviour principles

A child with a disability can present behaviours that are complex and difficult to understand, not only for parents but for extended family such as grandparents, siblings, aunts and uncles, and close friends. They may not have experienced these types of behaviours before and so will not understand them. This can create relationship difficulties and conflict if parents are given negative comments about their child along the lines of them 'just being naughty'. The learning and adjustments needed to be made by parents should be spread to the wider family support network. For example, it could be suggested that parents invite other family members or friends to attend parenting courses such as Triple P (many courses are available depending upon a child's disability) with them, or be at the family home when other agency professionals attend to advise and guide. This can be presented to the family as building a supportive foundation for the child's future and well-being.

A key point to remind parents of is that there can still be general behaviour management strategies, which are usually the main points of house rules and boundaries. The key message is to find ways in which to adapt the general rule to make it clear, understandable and achievable for their child's level of understanding and physical ability.

General behaviour management and house rules can look and be adapted like this:

» Parents wanting their child to sit down to eat can change the phrase to 'good sitting' when the child does sit down. This encourages even young toddlers to learn the good behaviour that earns them praise.

» If a parent is trying to get their child not to shout or be aggressive in their tone, they could give the message 'good talking with a thumbs up sign' to show when the volume of their voice is just right. Parents might need to be advised that if their child is shouting a good approach is to whisper back to them and bring the volume down themselves, as shouting or raising voices back at the child to ask them to be quiet will do the opposite.

» The general wearing of seatbelts in cars can become a battle, and the advice to share with parents is for them not to try and drive the car until the seatbelts are fastened. If they are undone during driving the car must be pulled up in a safe place; a really good approach is to remain quiet until the child asks why you have stopped. It can then be explained that you cannot drive until they are nice and safe with their seatbelt fastened. Also you need to get them to consider whereabouts the child is sitting in the car, especially if their behaviour is unpredictable.

» When a parent is trying to stop their child who has a learning disability with presenting behaviours such as slapping or hitting, you may find them using instructions such as 'stop slapping' or 'stop hitting'; unconsciously they are actually encouraging the behaviour to continue. This is because the negative words 'slapping' or 'hitting' can become trigger words, with the child hearing them as an instruction or action word. 'Stop' or 'don't' can for some children present as a dare or create an opportunity for defiance to test their boundaries. We can all recognise the phrase 'don't slam the door' – which is often followed by the door slamming. Parents can be advised to use the term 'kind hands' to a child with limited understanding. The term 'kind hands' needs to be accompanied by the parent taking a gentle hold of the child's hands and bringing them down by their side. A gentle stroke of their arm can demonstrate a kind touch to show the child what 'kind hands' feels like. Sentences beginning with 'stop' or 'don't' can be rephrased into positive suggestions such as 'play nicely', or 'be gentle with your sister' or 'thank you for closing the door nicely'.

» It is worth reminding parents that their children will do as they do: their child will take clues from them on how to behave in the world. They are their child's role model, and so they will need to demonstrate the rules they set themselves in order that they can guide by example. If parents want their child to say 'please', they need to say it in context themselves. If parents don't want their child to shout, they need to not shout themselves.

» Encouraging parents to spot good behaviours can be a rewarding approach for both them and their child. You might need to help them see the good things that are going unnoticed as the focus is on dealing with the difficult behaviours. For some children with very challenging behaviours this might need to start with the smallest thing they do that is good, such as hanging their coat up, putting something in the bin or sitting down for a couple of minutes. As a social worker when you visit you will be able to help parents find the good, and by pointing these out and encouraging parents to pounce on the positive they will begin to see this approach work.

» Whether the child is very young, a wheelchair user, or laid on a bed or the floor due to their physical disability, it is good practice for parents to be reminded to get down to their child's level. This helps the child engage and know that their parent is joining in their world to play, and even more importantly, enables the parents to have insight into the views and perspectives of their child. This can be quite enlightening, especially when a child is being taken out for a walk down the street in a pushchair or wheelchair. It is often taken for granted that as adults we can see over hedges and into gardens, and can see houses, trees, ponds and general things that are going on around the child. Getting down to their level in the street can show how their visibility is not as rich, as they may only be able to see the hedge and the sky: the houses will be behind the hedge or wall from their low-level eye perspective. It is a most valuable thing for parents to take a moment to stop and meet their child's eye level in lots of different environments so they can understand how their child is seeing the world.

Mapping resources within

Before looking at how parents can learn and develop strategies to manage their children's presenting challenges, it is worth noting that there will be parents who are first and foremost exhausted and exasperated by the high level of care, attention and supervision their child requires. In the first instance there may need to be opportunities to explore how the parents can re-charge from this daily high-level care. In terms of severe levels of disability and related challenging and physical behaviours, you may find parents who are quite isolated from their wider families for various reasons, and thus be reliant on authorities to provide respite services, which for some families can be a real identified need. You may also find that because of how services have been delivered to families in the recent past, there is an identified culture and belief in some parents that as they cannot manage their child's challenging behaviours the only option is to look at residential educational or respite settings – and they will fight for their believed right to have this service agreed and funded. For most families who are established and live within their own local community with their own family network around them or close by, however, you will find hidden resources within this network that is centred on the child. This can be seen as a family's 'wealth' in terms of having available support at various levels, from emotional and practical support to the children staying with family members or being taken out for a few hours by a trusted friend. One key approach here is to formulate a plan that lays out the support and respite provided for the family by the network of involved people, whereby parents are able to see the pressure shared out and their respite built into a plan of what would normally happen within close communities.

Very often you will find that parents feel they have no support until the plan is drawn up for them to highlight their supportive network. This approach also moves practice towards enabling families to draw upon their own resources and thus not need statutory involvement, the paradigm social work practice is moving toward. You will recognise this approach within the SOS model and in using Family Group Conferencing, among other strength-based, empowering and enabling approaches that are underpinned by the concept of families taking back their responsibilities for finding solutions and planning themselves to problem solve.

It is important to sit with parents and complete a genogram that gives them a visual view of their support networks, and also add to this the people who may not be family but who the child would say are important to them and who could help support them. Please see Chapter 6 for an example of a genogram.

Research has recognised that bringing the family network round the table to discuss support needs for the child they are related to brings a whole new meaning to family support plans. There is great value in recognising resources within families. In order to keep with the current trend of exploring family wealth in terms of support, it is good practice to discuss with parents who they will want to attend the review and planning meetings, and this does not necessarily mean agencies as it has done historically. If professionals do remain involved, however, you should consider if needs could be met through a Team Around the Child (TAC) rather than at a Child in Need level.

Social barriers and impact

For parents living with a child with a sensory processing disorder, ADHD or severe learning difficulties, there will be certain needs and considerations. Here are a few examples:

» The home may need to have security measures in place to protect the child. These will also restrict movements for family members as internal and external doors and windows need to be constantly locked.

» Parents may find that as part of their child's autism they need to learn to accept the responses they may or may not receive from their child when trying to show affection towards them. Other family members would need to learn to understand this.

» Some parents may find it difficult to understand or change their child's repeated or rigid behaviours and obsessions.

» Some parents may not be able to hug or hold their child due to the child's high sensory needs.

» There may be challenging behaviour to manage, and it can be difficult for parents to know how to effect change.

» A child with autism may want to be in control of their environment and find it difficult to let others into their world.

» Siblings may be rebelling and want to be able to follow their own agendas like their sibling does.

» There may be stressful and fractious relationships within the family.

» You may find exhausted, exasperated and stressed parents who are close to a family breakdown.

» In homes you may find walls scribbled on, wallpaper stripped off, doors and furniture broken or damaged or the home bare of ornaments and decorative pieces.

» Parents and family members 'treading on egg shells' in their own home to prevent outbursts and challenging behaviours.

» Families may not be able to attend social events and functions due to fear of outbursts of aggression, often leaving them socially isolated.

As a social worker in a children with disabilities team, you will be working with specialist educational and respite settings, where you will find different approaches used to support the children with their disability related needs. While it is good experience to see and develop the different approaches and techniques used by the different professionals and settings involved, you can find this may also present you with dilemmas and complicating factors as exampled in the case below.

Case study: Severe autism and aggression

Jamie is 17 and has severe autism and high sensory needs; he requires spinning and swinging movements and sensory experiences in order to reduce his anxieties. Jamie has a shared care arrangement with his respite setting and his home as he is a tall, well-framed young person who can display challenging, aggressive and physical outbursts if his anxieties are raised. There was an agreed plan to progress Jamie to the next steps toward independence given his age, to prepare him for moving on to adult services and further learning. He was given a larger bedroom and had teenage pictures hung, with new bedding and furnishings. The new room was close to the bathroom and it was planned that he would develop his independence and be more self-contained but still have support around him. This had been done in stages as it was understood that he does not accept change well and needed lots of time and preparation. Nevertheless, he tore down the pictures, pulled down the curtains, broke some of the furniture and began to display high levels of anxiety – resulting in hitting out at people.

Jamie was seen by his social worker on a visit, where he had been on his iPad looking at his favourite clips. It had been recognised that his favourite clip was from a classic children's cartoon and that he continued to repeat some of the short clips in order to hear the sounds he liked. He was seen as very relaxed and happy in doing this, as this activity was placing no demands upon him. It was recognised that at the age of 17 his emotional development age was very much at a toddler stage and so it became apparent that he was not yet at the developmental stage of moving toward independence and having so many changes and demands placed upon him.

This example has been shared to remind you that there will be challenges with schools, even specialist schools as in this example, due to their need to meet their performance targets and to take children through the school curriculum and academic year levels; it could be argued that the child would not cope at these levels by virtue of their own developmental stage, which is often much younger than their biological age. While it is sad to think about the slow pace of development that some young people with disabilities have, it needs to be recognised as equally important that each child is unique and will need to make slow, steady progress via small achievable tasks at their own developmental level and pace, and so arguably should not be pushed into fitting into peer group and curriculum levels based on their age alone.

Strategies, techniques and programmes to support

In Chapter 5 we introduced you to autism, giving you a whistle-stop tour of the triad of impairments identified when working with autistic children. As you will discover, when communication is impaired and the child cannot express their needs and wishes, this can result in challenging behaviours being displayed. Furthermore, when a child's parents or carers cannot understand their communication signs and behaviours, which are often a form of communication in themselves, this can heighten frustrations and create further negative behaviours. Most parents who are attending children's centres, special schools or child development centres are invited to attend courses and groups to help them learn about these behaviours and how to maximise support. They also offer opportunities to find peer support from other parents who share common ground. There are also charity websites and parent forums where parents can feel supported and share their experiences, trials and successes with others. You won't be expected to have all the answers and resolve parents' difficulties, but you can refer and pass on any relevant information you find in your research and reading.

Many children with complex learning disabilities or who are on the autistic spectrum are rigid in imagination and thoughts and not open to change. They become anxious, and need time to process change and warning of events that are going to happen or be different. They are often isolated, have a lack of empathy for other people's feelings and have difficulty in processing information. Children with autism need to socialise with other children but this must be done in a more gradual way, such as play with one child then increase this to two children, then to three etc over a slow period. Placing a child with autism into a large group such as a toddler group or after-school club would be too overpowering and for some can create an information overload. Autistic children need time to adjust to their environments.

As with most general approaches to behaviour management, the key is in finding the positives, interests and strengths of the child that can be built upon. Rather than looking at unwanted behaviours as a strategy, a more positive approach is to look at what children are good at and what they like doing. Especially in children with disabilities, they can and do learn from receiving praise and positive reactions to even the smallest positive action. Sometimes parents might need to be reminded of the tiny positives that have become lost in their daily challenges.

For a child who has a sensory processing disorder, you may find parents talking about daily battles in trying to get their child to school on time. This can provide a useful opportunity to demonstrate to parents how their child can become distressed with information overload, when they think they are just instructing their child to get ready.

Activity: **Keeping it simple**

Jason's mother is trying to get him to get ready to leave for school:

1. *'Get your coat on, Jason'*

2. *'Jason, hurry up and get your coat on'*

3. *'Come on Jason, hurry up, you'll be late for school'*

4. *'Oh for goodness' sake Jason, what have I told you? Why haven't you got your coat on yet?'*

5. *'Right Jason, that's it, I am cross with you now, you never do as you're told, just do as I tell you will you?'*

The five sentences above show how the instructions given to Jason have quickly gone from five words to 24 words, and the final sentence does not contain the original request. The child is overloaded as he cannot process all the information at the same time.

Twenty seconds is an approximate timeframe for some children with additional needs to process the first instruction. If more information is given before this time lapses then the processing time needs to begin again. If the instruction needs to be given again, parents need to try and repeat the same first simple instruction without adding any new words. This would help reduce behaviours and battles in the mornings; the key piece of advice for parents is to allow time and to be patient.

Drawing on strengths

Some children with additional needs, in particular with autism, may present with particular skills and talents that make it difficult for their parents to understand how their child can have high levels of intelligence in some areas and low emotional and social development and understanding in others, those that create their challenging behaviours. These developed abilities can be recognised as 'autistic savant', a condition in which special, occasionally outstanding, talents exist in individuals with otherwise moderate or profound learning difficulties (see the film *Rain Man* for a portrayal of an autistic savant).

The talents tend to be in the area of music, calendar calculation, maths or drawing. To a parent or onlooker the child can appear to be obsessed or repeating behaviours like opening and shutting doors and locks, or listening to or watching just one part of a video or cartoon; this repeated behaviour, with the other sensory feedback it gives to the child, makes them feel safe and in control. It is how this is managed and balanced with the child that parents will need support with, as well as developing their understanding about these behaviours. One example is a young boy who only wants to talk about trains and tunnels: in order that his mother could get him to talk about other things like what he would like for tea, or where they were going when they went out, they had a scheme of taking turns – mum asks a question, he gives an answer and *then* he can tell her a fact about a train or tunnel.

This can become exhausting and relentless but it is something that some parents need to do to create a balance and reduce their child's obsessive and repetitive behaviours.

Some special abilities that have been reported include:

» exceptional drawing abilities

» high proficiency at playing a musical instrument or even composing music

» performing lengthy numerical calculations, such as doing square roots on huge numbers

» identifying the days of the week on which any date fell or will fall in a wide span of years, commonly known as calendar calculation

» reading fluently at a very young age though not necessarily comprehending the text well

» memorising huge amounts of facts about favourite subjects

» dismantling and reassembling complex machines, such as radios

» working with computers

In order for parents to help their child make the world less confusing, they need to develop routines and structures that their child can feel safe with, for example, always walking the same route to school. In class, they may get upset if there is a sudden change to the timetable. Some children may need to be allowed into the classroom earlier so they are already in class when the other children arrive; this would be because the child is unable to enter a room that is already full of children.

Children with Asperger's syndrome often prefer to order their day to a set pattern. For example, if they travel to school at set times in the day, an unexpected delay to their journey to or from school can make them anxious or upset. A main characteristic of Asperger's is that young people can struggle to make and maintain friendships, as they don't understand the unwritten social rules that most of us pick up without thinking. For example, they may stand too close to another person, or start an inappropriate topic of conversation and find other people unpredictable and confusing. They may become withdrawn and seem uninterested in other people, appearing almost aloof or as behaving in what may seem like an inappropriate manner.

To look at some real examples of how and why routines and structure are important for some young people with Asperger's, with some having a real need to have a strict and detailed timetable of events, it is worth reading *The Curious incident of the Dog in the Night-Time* by Mark Haddon. This demonstrates how this daily routine is a high need in terms of knowing what the day is going to look like.

'Theory of Mind' by Simon Baron-Cohen (1994) explains how children with autism may have difficulty in understanding others' behaviour.

A psychological theory of autism, the 'theory of mind' hypothesis, claims that children with autism fail to develop the ability to think about mental states in the normal way, and thus fail to understand behaviour in terms of mental states.

(Baron-Cohen et al 1994: 515)

Here is our interpretation of what this means in example terms.

» Global developmental delay or autism impairs a child's ability to use their imagination, which means it is difficult to role play or play pretend games, for example: pretending to have a steering wheel and that you are driving a bus; or putting a blanket over a table and playing at being in a tent or a cave. To some children with learning difficulties and cognitive impairment, the table remains a table and being sat under it would literally mean that they are sat under a table; in general, pretend and imaginative play is a difficult concept.

» When there is a problem to solve we generally weigh up the options and consequences and are able to make an informed decision based on our thought processing and being able to predict the consequences of the various options. Some children with learning difficulties and/or cognitive processing disorders may be unable to have this level of problem solving, especially if the problem is new or unexpected. Being able to see consequences and visualise outcomes of events are difficult because their thought processes are slowed and impaired. Without this ability to use thought processing to problem solve, we would often see anxiety raised in the children. For some children with severe autism or high levels of anxieties this could present as going into crisis and becoming distraught, and they may often display aggressive outbursts of challenging and physical behaviours.

» Children with learning disabilities do not always see danger, as they may not be able to think things through or to predict a safe outcome for themselves. For example, when crossing the road, there is no concept of looking or checking for traffic and most will often just step out onto the road without any awareness of oncoming traffic or the dangers present. If the park with swings is on the other side of the road, this will be their only focus, so they will need closely supervising and holding safely across the road. One autistic boy had a fascination with the sea at the beach and would literally keep walking out into the sea if left unsupervised, without any awareness of the cold or the dangers of the sea in general.

CAMHS as a key partner

As a social worker being involved with children with disabilities, you will find that there are key professional agencies that can support you as well as families directly. Children with disabilities often present with additional, related factors that affect their emotional health and well-being. Sensory processing, anxiety related behaviours and social or communication difficulties are a few examples of where specialist and psychological input and support are necessary. For many years previously, families struggled to understand why their child was behaving in certain ways and to know how to help them. Not so many years ago, young children were placed in institutions due to their mental health-related behaviours, which are now recognised as them being on the autistic spectrum or having attachment difficulties or ADHD. Sometimes their conditions were misdiagnosed due to the presence of a set of common symptoms. These were children who needed their families close by, supporting them and keeping them at home. To meet the gap identified by the children's National Service Framework (2004) regarding Child and Adolescent Mental Health Service (CAMHS) services for children with disabilities, by extending and improving access to CAMHS for these children and their families, NICE (The National Institute for Health and Care Excellence) produced some specific guidance around the management of autism in children and young people.

www.nice.org.uk/sharedlearning/the-behaviour-and-family-support-team-a-specialist-child-and-adolescent-mental-health-service-for-children-with-disabilities-and-their-families

While individual CAMHS teams across the country may have their own referral criteria and areas of focus, they mostly provide assessment and interventions for children and young people aged up to 18 who have an autism spectrum diagnosis, severe learning disabilities or complex physical and sensory disabilities. Interventions often focus on challenging behaviour or mental health difficulties that are related to the disability. From the authors' experience, however, there are times when it can be difficult to distinguish if a child's problems are related to their learning difficulties or mental health, particularly when they are displaying aggressive behaviour. Although social workers look to a social model to manage a child's disability and behaviours, sometimes we do need to explore the medical model to maintain the equilibrium and settle the child, in order to maintain the placement at home and stop a family breakdown. It can be very challenging if CAMHS and social care do not agree, CAMHS will not prescribe medication, the social worker has exhausted other avenues and the family are at crisis. This is the type of situation you will have to manage.

In children who have presented with specific behaviours, CAMHS have been known to make observations of the child or give advice and guidance based on the information that is shared. Some real examples of actual strategies shared below show how CAMHS have supported and advised either directly with a parent or indirectly through a social worker:

» *My son Luke keeps laying heavily on me and wanting to hug me tight all the time. He has classic autism and it is difficult to negotiate with him to give me some space.* It was suggested by a CAMHS psychologist that Luke is sensory seeking and needing pressure as this is often something that accompanies sensory processing difficulties (you might want to read more about 'sensory diets'). Mum was advised to build some hugs into his schedule so he can learn to receive the hugs following an activity or a task. Luke can learn that he will get the pressure hugs but not randomly and not by demand. Mum was also advised to purchase a gym ball that would allow Luke to roll about on the ball and receive the pressure and sensory motion that he is seeking. This worked well for Luke and the gym ball became a permanent fixture in the sitting room.

» *My son Christian gets anxious and angry when waiting for appointments and in leaving the house to go for them as they are not part of his routine.* Mum was advised by CAMHS to use picture symbols to show the car, and a picture of the hospital and one of home, so he could know the sequence of events and places and will know that he will be going home after the hospital. Mum had taken this and added her idea of laminating a white sheet of paper with a red cross in the middle as this way it suited any appointments that were held at the hospital.

» *My daughter Stacey has severe autism and will slap me hard. The more I tell her not to do that she will keep on slapping and it hurts as she is a strong girl getting bigger.* Mum was advised by CAMHS that as speech is not available to Stacey, her slapping would be a form of communication and a way of her expressing herself. Mum was advised to pass a cushion to Stacey to hold, which would give her hands something to hold and thus stop her need to slap. With this action repeated each time the slapping was about to happen, Stacey learned over time to grab a cushion herself when she needed to slap and slapped the cushion instead.

There are some young people with disabilities who are also suffering with mental health problems. For example Amy had Down's syndrome and low cognitive ability but was reaching the age of 16 years. Amy presented with hearing voices and having visions of people who she believed were telling her to do bad things. This had created a real worry as she actually jumped down the stairs as she thought she had been told to jump. This raised questions and discourse around medication or therapy and it wasn't until the therapy intervention was seen not to be working and Amy had more incidents that put her at risk of self-harm that appropriate medication was prescribed. It had been identified that medication needed to work alongside other therapies in order for the intervention to help Amy change her behaviour. In situations like this you will be involved in a Care Plan Approach (CPA) and you may be involved in making decisions around mental health capacity, which is discussed more in Chapter 1.

Building a positive working relationship with the CAMHS service and psychologists will be a valuable asset to you in your work and in accessing support and guidance for the families you will work with. CAMHS will have varying levels of criteria across the different authorities, but they have child and adolescent mental health as a focus and you will come across young people with Asperger's and severe autism whose emotional needs and mental health are affected by their disability and so may fit into the criteria for CAMHS support and services.

Risk assessing and family safety planning

Let's have a look at a case example activity around risks associated with challenging behaviours to begin developing your thoughts around support strategies and approaches to minimise or manage risk.

Activity: **Behaviour challenges**

Freddy's mum Sarah cannot take him out in the community alone as he has unpredictable outbursts that often lead to physical aggression, which Sarah cannot manage now Freddy is taller and much bigger than her. This leaves mum isolated at home when Freddy is not at school as dad Andy works away most of the time. Freddy attends a specialist education setting, but only for two mornings per week.

Can you imagine how it is for Freddy's mother? Can you think of areas where this pressure could be taken from her? Who else is in this? Can school do any more to help?

Below is a simple example of a risk assessment using plain and clear terminology that can be used with parents in looking at risks and prevention at home and in the community. The example can be adapted to suit any eventuality and expanded to include more detail where needed. You will become familiar with risk assessments. For example, you may be asked to help a family undertake a risk assessment in terms of setting up a direct payment support plan where they will be employing a support person who will need a thoroughly thought out risk assessment to ensure the child's safety while in their care. There is a website about direct payments that has risk assessment templates which can be used in relation to risk planning when support is funded through direct payments. We have included a link at the end of this chapter for you to take this further if needed.

Take a look at this activity to get you started!

Activity: **Talking about safety and risks**

Scenario: Just taking Simon to the shops in the car is very difficult for his mum and dad, as he will run off in the car park if given the chance. He is autistic and if he sees a green car he needs to run and chase after it, as he likes green things and he likes cars, so when there is a green car he just dashes off. He has no awareness of the dangers and of the car manoeuvring. Mum also has a young baby so it is very difficult for her to manage both Simon and the baby.

Activity/event	What harm might happen?	How can this risk be reduced?
Shopping trip	Simon may run off in the car park and get injured by a car manoeuvring.	Keep the child lock on to ensure Simon cannot just exit the car on his own.
		Keep Simon in the car until baby is fastened into the shopping trolley.
		If necessary use reins to securely hold Simon while he transitions from car to the shop.
		Give Simon a picture of a green car or a toy car so he can focus on these in his hands to distract him from looking for other cars.

These are just a few ideas, and it would be good practice to create the risk assessment in conversation with parents and family members in order to get them thinking of ways in which they can reduce risks and plan ahead for events such as trips out in busy places, or events that may present with hazards such as lakes, beaches, bus stations etc.

Now write a simple risk assessment for David's situation. See what ideas you can come up with to reduce risks for David.

Activity: **David**

Scenario: David has no awareness of danger and will try and run out of the house if left unsupervised. David will bite his hand, smear after going to the toilet etc if he is not supervised. David has no sense of pain or hot or cold water so he would not know if he has hurt himself and thus needs constant supervision to keep him safe from harm.

Again just having conversations with parents and laying out the risks in front of them in this way enables them to plan and think about the risks and how they can be managed and reduced. It is an honest and open approach to express your worries so that parents can have the opportunity to consider them and how they need to address the concerns and make their plans for safety.

There may be times when you find as in other social work disciplines that there are worries around risk which you feel that parents are not addressing effectively. Or it may be that you find parents at a low ebb in their situation, and they have lost their motivation to make the changes necessary to reduce the risks presented.

As with most behaviour related situations, parents can find themselves stuck at trying to prevent their child from having aggressive outbursts, so they allow them to develop a level of control and then the parents can find themselves too far down this path to regain parental control. The authors have experienced families treading on eggshells with their children holding all the power and even controlling what their parents can and cannot do. We have seen phones ripped out of sockets or smashed to prevent parents talking to people outside the home about their situation. These parents will need support to regain their parental control, either by referring to services that can provide this or by you as their social worker undertaking some direct work with the family.

Taking it further

Family Group Conference – Family Rights Group – Keeping Children Safe in their Families

www.frg.org.uk/involving-families/family-group-conferences

Haddon, M (2004) *The Curious Incident of the Dog in the Night-Time*. London: Vintage Publishing. Page 192 will show you a good example of a rigid routine timetable of a typical day that shows the attention to detail minute by minute, which was important for the author at the time the book was written.

The Signs of Safety is an innovative strengths-based, safety-organised approach to child protection casework, created by Andrew Turnell and Steve Edwards. The approach can be used in other areas where there are worries to be considered. In working with children with disabilities, this approach can be used with family to enable them to understand, plan and reduce the worries and risks presented in caring for the child and keep them safe from harm. This approach can help to develop your risk assessment planning with families in a way that balances the family's strengths and resources while considering what needs to happen to reduce or remove the worries and risks. Find out more by using the link to the website.

Signs of Safety www.signsofsafety.net/

Triple P is a positive parenting programme based on evidence. Triple P gives parents simple and practical strategies to help them confidently manage their children's behaviour, prevent problems developing and build strong, healthy relationships. In looking at further strategies to support children with disabilities, this book offers an array of guidance, tools and templates that you can use with families:

Sanders, M R, Massucchelli, T G and Studman, L J (2003) *Stepping Stones Triple P: For Families with a Child Who Has a Disability: Family Work Book* (Edition 2). Brisbane: The University of Queensland and Disability Services.

The Children's Sleep Charity works to ensure children get a good night's sleep – and thus so do their parents. www.thechildrenssleepcharity.org.uk.

Direct Payment - Risk Assessments

www.hse.gov.uk/healthservices/direct-payments.hgm

Chapter 8 | Giving consideration to values, ethics, race and anti-discriminatory practice

This chapter includes a case study and discusses a range of ethical issues, discrimination and varying value-based thinking. It explores issues associated with the child's ethnicity and/or race and their disability, with some challenges that can be presented within personal or professional boundaries. This chapter guides you towards promoting disability in a positive light, through creating opportunities to develop a wider insight into some of the barriers children with disabilities face within the community and society in general.

This is your personal opportunity to be honest with yourself about how the presenting issues make you feel, and how you might approach similar challenges in the future. You are allowed to feel awkward, annoyed, angry, frustrated, shocked, hopeful, creative or anything else – you just need to listen to the values from within, hear what they are saying to you, note them down and let them out!

Equality and access

The word 'disabled', if taken apart and critically examined, shows how society had historically created a culture with public amenities whereby there was a 'norm' in terms of people who can walk, see, hear and talk having the ultimate access to social activities and public places. Houses, shops and buildings were built with appliances and equipment that were difficult to access by a 'disabled' person: concrete steps, revolving doors, public transport etc. Society had unconsciously put up the barriers that meant that a person with a disability was 'disabled' by society itself. Historically, society has ensured that people with a disability have had to fit into the societal norm, leading to discrimination, labelling and segregation within communities.

Think about the phrase 'disabled person' and now think about the phrase 'person with a disability'. The second phrase sees and acknowledges the person before the disability. In 1995 the Disability Discrimination Act was introduced by the government to protect and promote the rights of 'disabled people' and to make it unlawful to discriminate against them. The Act was produced after much consultation with and feedback from disability rights groups, and aims to ensure that they are treated equally by employers and service providers. In 2005 the Act was amended with the aim of ending disability-related harassment. The legislation was extended, with core additions covering public transport for disabled people as well as access to premises and private clubs. It reaffirmed its commitment to end the ignorance, thoughtlessness and prejudice that affected the lives of certain disadvantaged people.

Life was very difficult at one time for people with disabilities and their families, and while there has been great movement in striving for equality and access there remains a journey ahead with many more changes in policies, and more importantly in attitudes, to come. A whole change in mind-set is needed and as we know this does not happen over the short term. Even in our new legislation you will read the term 'disabled people' used when describing how policies are moving to help. If we can speak on behalf of people with disabilities, it is not help that is needed in policy: it is equality and recognition of the person first. It is not about 'doing a favour', it is about making access equal for all. It seems that there is a way to go until a wheelchair sign no longer needs displaying over an adapted toilet in a public place. One day all toilets will be built equally sized and equipped to ensure that everyone has full access, without segregation.

In 2006 the government introduced the Disability Equality Duty, specifically aimed at the public sector. It encourages local authorities, hospitals, schools and colleges etc to publish a report to explain their progress in promoting equality and detail what action they are taking in practical steps to meet the needs of disabled people. The Equality and Human Rights Commission took over the duties of The Disability Rights Commission when it closed down in 2007.

There is an example below of how the government are trying to get it right with their strategy leading up to 2025, starting by setting up an Office for Disability Issues (ODI) to try to help the public sector and central government to improve the delivery of facilities to disabled people. One of its key objectives is to ensure that by 2025 anyone with a disability will have the same opportunities in their work and social lives as the rest of the United Kingdom's population. As you can read in their statement, while they have referred to people with a disability having the same opportunities, they have also referred to the delivery of better facilities to 'disabled people': www.officefordisability.gov.uk.

A report called *Improving the Life Chances of Disabled People* was written by the ODI in consultation with disability rights groups. The document highlights the challenges that those with disabilities need to overcome, and states that people from all sections of British social life have a part to play in helping to tackle prejudice. The ODI acknowledges that everyday tasks like shopping, going to the cinema or applying for a job can present many difficulties for people with disabilities and that this is related to attitudinal, cultural and societal barriers that are long recognised to be a uphill struggle to overcome.

A different kind of rational thinking, such as the application of the social model of disability, brings a different perspective; a model that requires change from the world to socially 'include' the individual, challenging oppression and discrimination implicit in both individual and medical model approaches, especially in relation to cultural and structural levels (Thompson, 2006:25).

You will need to develop the ability to challenge some prejudices and advocate for the empowerment of children you will work with, which will require a great deal of your rational knowledge and understanding. *'It requires knowledge that can…[examine social structures and systems]… focus on a strengths perspective whilst considering the capacities and potentialities of the user with particular emphasis on respect and service user determination'* (Healy, 2005:151–152). It will be a great skill for you as a social worker to promote the involvement, voice and views of the child using practised methods of appropriate communication (see Chapter 4).

Positive rephrasing

You may have read some previous Special Educational Needs Statements and seen the difficulties presented with them. For example: 'Jonny is unable to walk for more than 20 steps and will need a rollator to help him' or 'Lucy is unable to wash and clean herself after she has visited the toilet'. The words unable or cannot appear as a first introduction of a skill that is difficult, making it a negative statement. It is difficult for parents to have to read a list of negative statements about their child, and this often colours the parents and professionals' expectations of the child's level of ability or their disability. There is a way of turning the negative comments around so that they still explain the child's need for support, but use positive, strengths-based statements to recognise a 'can do' approach with regard to a child's abilities. Let's look at the first sentence again and rephrase it, perhaps to say:

Jonny can walk for about 10 steps on his own before he then needs the rollator to help with further steps. With support and encouragement he can develop to increase the number of steps possible as his muscles and balance strengthen.

Let's try rephrasing the second sentence:

Lucy can take herself to the toilet and will let the teacher know when she is finished and will then need support to help her clean herself properly, as she is trying to do as much as she can herself and will learn more steps at her own pace, with encouragement and support.

Try having a look at some reports that have been written by other people or agencies who have used a focus on what the child cannot do and see how you can change the wording to promote a 'can do' style. This is not to be critical of previous practice but a way of examining how you can strive towards making positive changes for the future.

Perhaps you will find yourself at a meeting where professionals reflect or report on the difficult tasks that the child is unable to do. You can use rephrasing in your reviewing questions to identify more about the abilities of the child, and furthermore, you can begin to write the review or a new plan for the child by using positive 'can do' statements. This can be a small seed of change that will grow and you will see other professionals (though not all) picking up the new terminology that promotes the strengths and abilities of the child. This positive approach is beginning to show through in the new Education, Health and Care Plans, where the focus is on what outcomes from intervention or support will be achieved, using terms like 'will be able to' or 'will be enjoying' to reflect the positive outcome for the child.

You may hear parents describing to you what their child cannot do in relation to their disability, whether this is due to them hearing these messages from medical or other professionals or them just having fallen into the trap of not being able to recognise the positive aspects of their child's abilities. It would be part of your role to advocate the child's strengths and abilities to their parents or carers. For example, a mother has informed you that her son Jack cannot use a knife or fork and cannot feed himself. You observe that Jack has global development delay, which for him means he is operating at a toddler age rather than his physical age of six. You highlight to his mother that he can feed himself if he uses his fingers, and could remind her that this is appropriate for his age of development. You will need to be able to identify the smallest of positives and abilities in order to help the parent see and identify them, and this positive outlook will grow on them too.

Rephrasing sounds like a small action and you might question what it has to do with discrimination and values? Well, consider that when reports are written about a child this information follows them through their education and later on into their young adult life. This influences the care and support they receive from their carers, and moreover, how the carers respond and approach their care – based on the information presented about the child or young person. If children continue to have reports and statements of what they *cannot* do as the main focus, they can become labelled or segregated and in some cases will not be encouraged to aspire to try to achieve new things by their carers. This can lead carers to discriminate by omission and create oppression in the carer's approach and care.

How often have we seen carers continuing to care for a young person in the way that they have been advised from reports or statements as there have been few expectations placed on the young person's abilities? The young person is at risk of becoming stuck at this stage of development unless someone is brave enough to stop and take a 'can do' approach, which will enable them to build on their strengths and skills. The authors have experienced some parents accepting their child's inabilities as written on their statements as a 'statement of fact'; for example, if it states that their child cannot use a knife or fork to eat, some parents have continued to just feed their child themselves, even as they grow, as they feel that there is nothing to gain and so do not attempt to teach the child to feed themselves. Not dissimilar is how some parents will not feed a child certain foods because at their first taste they did not like it and would not eat it. The food item becomes written off the child's menu for good and is not introduced to the child to give it another try. Parents will view their child as a faddy eater, which becomes an accepted fact with the child confirming this as a self-fulfilling prophecy. It might take a lot longer to achieve a child being able to move and progress with certain things, and it will need step-by-step approaches with lots of encouragement and praise to see skills achieved. The most important aspect here is that the child needs to be valued and given worth by having this time and patience invested in them.

Influential recording

Some parents take written statements and reports with the professional credibility they are worth, so when writing reports yourself be mindful of the messages you are sending out about the child's potential. Remember how influential your information is in the child's future progress and how it may affect their care and support and attitudes they receive. While trying to balance their needs for support, keep in mind their individuality, strengths and can do's and try not to use stereotypical or labelling statements that could begin their journey of discrimination and segregation; remember, keep to the facts.

One example of this is the term global developmental delay (GDD), which often accompanies other disabilities or conditions and means that all aspects of development, such as walking, speech and learning, have been delayed in some way. It is helpful to understand that GDD will affect each child differently, so it would be good practice to describe more specifically how their GDD manifests itself. Remember to keep the statements strength based. For example: *'Alfie has global developmental delay, which means for him that while he is able to walk, he remains unsteady and requires support with something to hold on to or his rollator. He is able to ask for things using one or two words, like "me drink", and is able to know when he is having a wee in his nappy by tapping his nappy to show you.'*

Voice and views of the child

One of the biggest critiques of case recording in our experience that has been raised many times by Ofsted and auditors is recording the child's voice. Many recordings have shown previous statements such as *'Jeremy is unable to share his views by virtue of his disability.'* This is no longer acceptable and you will be expected to find ways of ascertaining the voice of a child with a disability who does not have speech to communicate with. You are their advocate and they need you to learn how they communicate and express their needs, whether they make noises to show they are sad or happy, or clap their hands or bang their arms on their chest to show their excitement, or rock back and forth when they are anxious (see Chapter 4).

Close observation is needed when working with a child or young person with a disability. They may turn their head away from a carer when they enter a room and this could easily be missed if you are not watching closely. You may need to visit more regularly so you can learn their patterns of behaviours and responses to people, and see their reactions to various situations and at different times of the day. This will help you know if they show changed responses to indicate any worries in relation to associated people or other things like the environment, which might trigger a facial expression that tells how they are feeling. The message is: don't assume that just because a child or young person cannot speak that they have nothing to say. Recognise and acknowledge them as a person first, learn how to listen to and understand them – value and respect must be first and foremost.

Inclusion

Sadly, there are still some people who see a child in a wheelchair and presume they have no voice, views or understanding. They will not engage with the child directly and some will not even look at them. Some people will have conversations with the carer or parent, either over the young person's head or by standing behind them so that they are not able to be part of the interaction and conversation. There are some carers who have been seen having conversations about the person in the wheelchair while ignoring or not even acknowledging that person. The authors have heard statements concerning children such as 'Does he like chocolate?', 'Oh, can she manage OK at school?' and 'What is her favourite music?' When the child or young person tries to respond and join in but has slowed or slurred speech, some people will try and finish their sentence or words for them rather than show the patience needed to allow them to finish what they are saying.

Fear of the unknown

There are some people who because they have never known anyone with a disability, actually fear the concept of disability and will avoid contact with people in wheelchairs or with a physical disability, or alternatively will be fascinated and stare. This demonstrates how society remains in its infancy in terms of understanding and respecting that these are children and people first, with views, ideas, intelligence and rights to be an equal part of society without discrimination, segregation or being stereotyped by people who do not understand or are just ignorant.

Double discrimination

Children and their families can face discrimination when their child has a disability; however when the child is also from a family who do not have English as a first language, and they have a 'different' cultural identity, they can be presented with double discrimination.

If you imagine all the words and terms used in this book in relation to disability and complex health issues, and then the medical terms for diagnosing conditions, medications and treatments. Now include talks of care plans, Child in Need plans, legislation around looked-after children or short breaks regulations. Both authors found as you may too that at the beginning of our journeys in working with children with disabilities it was like learning a new language.

Now consider being a parent living in this country whose first language is not English. Imagine that you are facilitating a CIN meeting with parents who are Polish and only settled in the country six months ago. They have come here to get better care for their child who has a physical disability and requires a new wheelchair: the one he has currently is too small and he cries in pain as the sides are digging into his thighs and making them sore. His parents do not know where to begin to look for support with this or which services can help.

From experience even interpreters can struggle to know some of the medical terms and language used. Even when you think you have covered everything by having an interpreter present, there needs to be lots of consideration of pace, with people speaking one at a time and also only sharing one sentence at a time so that the interpreter can translate each bit of information. If it would normally take an hour for a meeting, you need to allow at least two in these circumstances, especially if the parents are expected to read documents and also have their views and responses translated in the meeting.

At many meetings people want to chip in and share their thoughts on a subject, even with a fairly strict chairperson present. This can mean that parents miss out on chunks of views and information as the whole of the discussion has not been interpreted. This is discriminatory and excludes parents from partaking fully in the meeting. It is not usually done with intent, but happens when a group of professionals have become accustomed to talking amongst themselves at meetings: they will need pulling up as soon as it starts to happen so that the situation does not deteriorate. You may need to help the chair stop people talking over one another to ensure that no information is missed for the family.

There are other areas where the cultural diversity of families may present ethical and value-based issues. This case study is based on real experience but with the names and features of the situation changed.

Case study: Simmy

Simmy was born in Iran and has severe learning disabilities with no speech. He is 15 years old and had to become looked after due to his challenging behaviours. Simmy's family were Muslim and so his care plan had to include and consider his dietary needs, traditional festivals, personal care and his environment.

Simmy's mum Senab had attended his care setting and on one particular day had stayed until she had seen him and supported him in having his tea, then his bath and getting ready for bed. It had been discovered by staff the next morning when Simmy was being supported in the bathroom that he had had all his body hair shaved off, including from his arm pits and genital area. Staff had raised questions to the social worker around the appropriateness of a mother providing this kind of personal care to a 15-year-old son. Nikki the social worker had discussed the issue with her manager and also had a conversation with the safeguarding LADO to query whether this would be considered a safeguarding issue. At the same time Nikki did some research to see if this act was cultural and a part of the family's faith and religious needs. An article was found which explained that in the Muslim faith pubic hair is seen to be unclean and unhygienic and therefore all pubic hair is removed as part of a cleansing ritual.

This situation had caused lots of debates and received varying views from the staff and professionals involved. One male member of the residential staff had stated that even if he was asked to undertake this task, he would not want to as he felt it was 'too personal and not appropriate and also not seen as a basic need'. *The views of different colleagues varied from safeguarding matters around Senab not being open and honest about her intentions to provide this particular care and the appropriateness of her actions, to others that tried to factor in values and ethical or biased judgments. A safeguarding officer asked,* 'Would we be worried if it was a 15-year-old girl with a disability whose mother was tending to her personal care during her menstruation? No, we wouldn't in general, so why is it that we jumped to negative views when it is a mother tending to a personal care need of her son?'

Rather than jumping to the safeguarding procedures, in the first instance Nikki had been advised to have a conversation with Simmy's mother and father to explore with them if this action from Senab was part of their cultural beliefs and to also ask why and if it needs to be Senab performing this particular task.

Nikki had to use tact and diplomacy in approaching this sensitive subject with Senab and Rajid (father). Nikki had gone with some other issues to discuss and had also had some light conversation with Senab and Rajid as she needed to find the right moment. She began with, 'Well, now that's most of the things covered that we needed to discuss, but there is one more issue that I need to discuss with you that is a bit sensitive. I need to talk to you about how staff had noticed how Simmy had appeared in the bathroom the other morning with his pubic hair shaved off, and as Simmy cannot speak it can only be presumed that it was you, Senab, who did this when you visited the other night and stayed to bathe him?' *Senab agreed that she had done this and both Senab and Rajid smiled and agreed that it was a sensitive thing to discuss. Nikki asked* 'Is this part of your cultural belief to do this as I have read an article that does say that the Muslim faith see pubic hair as unhygienic?' *Rajid answered* 'Yes that is the case but we do this mainly to keep Simmy clean.' *Nikki asked* 'Is this something that needs to be performed by mothers only?' *Senab explained,* 'No, it is just that as Simmy is still needing to wear nappies and the weather has been very hot, I would not want to think that he has soiled and it gets left in his pubic hair, which could cause him to get sore or get an infection. I wanted to ensure that he could be kept clean underneath his nappy and as his mum I am more patient and will do the job properly for him.'

Both Senab and Rajid understood the dilemma that this action had caused and they both agreed that from then on Rajid will perform this care for Simmy – but he had to promise Senab that he would be patient and do a proper job.

This case generated some conversations about how professionals would approach issues like these from different perspectives, as when considering situations and family matters we all bring with us our own value base built on our own life experiences and religious, ethnic or cultural beliefs. Sheppard (1995:25–3) suggests that practice wisdom requires three types of knowledge: 'knowledge gained from everyday life', derived from the processes of living in society and interacting with others; 'knowledge gained from social science', specifically research and ideas; and 'knowledge gained from the conduct of social work practice'. The most important aspect of this case is how Nikki had taken a step back, had conversations with various people and most importantly taken some time to research the family's religion and culture, which helped her to understand that this particular personal care was for them borne out of the need for a high standard of hygiene and cleanliness. Nikki had also sensitively yet openly explored with the parents why they had a need to carry out this particular act on their son. With the approach she used, neither parent had been offended by the questions or conversations that followed, and instead they had been able to explore this care with Nikki to find the appropriate compromise.

It needs to be noted here that the outcome and management of this situation is not a written prescription for how this situation should have been managed, and there would be many other professionals who would most likely have made different but equally effective approaches. This case study has been provided as just one example with the salient point being that to understand something you need to have open and honest conversations about why you are asking and what the worry is, and to research and look to theories that help you understand.

As social work raises numerous questions, as a social worker you need a variety of possible answers or theories to make sense of the situations you are faced with. '*An important characteristic of a theory is that it goes beyond the descriptive to include explanations of why things happen in a given situation and can therefore guide you in decision making*' (Trevithick. 2006: 26). Here is an activity to enable your thoughts and considerations about different situations around this case study.

Activity: **Personal care and culture**

» *Is there anything in Simmy's case that you would have approached differently? If so, explain what the issues are and why.*

» *Can you think of other situations where there need to be considerations made around personal care and cultural needs? How would you approach these?*

> » *Perhaps you may find a child needing respite care who has thick afro hair; what care and consideration would this need?*

> » *Would you consider it appropriate for a father to attend to the personal and menstrual care of his 13-year-old daughter with a physical disability? Before answering a yes or no, consider the same question in different contexts; for example, is the father on his own as a single carer without family support?*

> » *As Simmy has no speech, the case has not been looked at from his perspective.*

>> » *What would this situation look and feel like for Simmy?*

>> » *How could you advocate his views and wishes about his personal care?*

> » *Consider what your own values are, and where they have come from.*

You might want to use the questions in this activity to share discussions with colleagues, friends and team members. This becomes more interesting when you include health and education professionals as they will also add their professional perspectives, like educational considerations or the medical model approach to care. You may find it interesting to hear the debates created by the subject and the different values you will find in different people. Remember that they each bring with them their own life experiences, beliefs and culture. It will help you to consider different perspectives and values along with your own, which will form the basis of your professional practice wisdom and knowledge.

Cultural care and law

In considering the case study further, the Children Act 1989 Section 22 5(C) requires that when making any decision about a child, the local authority must give *'due consideration to the child's religious persuasion, racial origin, culture and language'*. The new duty combines with another new duty to ensure that when children have to live away from their natural families, the local authority should also take steps to reunite such children with their families and to promote contact with the family during separation. These provisions should ensure that the specific needs of Asian children with disabilities are more precisely assessed and effectively met through a range of local services in the future. They set out specific duties for health authorities with regard to children in care for short- or long-term periods, which require them to be sensitive and responsive to the following areas:

> » The young person's perception of his or her health needs or disability.

> » The rationale of any treatment.

» The implications of care for the life of the family.

» The management of treatment or medication within the care setting.

» Any special areas of concern like sexuality, substance misuse, mental health problems or HIV infection (where confidentiality may be an issue).

» Counselling – for example on the implications of a condition like muscular dystrophy, which may only start to affect everyday life in early adolescence.

» The provision of aids and equipment.

» Purchasing arrangements for specialist healthcare when a child or young person is placed out of his or her health authority of origin.

» The interplay of ethnicity, religion, culture and language and how these affect all of the above.

Research undertaken for the Department for Education and Skills Market Research in 2006 shows that Asian families and children are considerably more likely to require disability support services, and they appear to receive atypical lower-cost services. More than one-fifth of the Asian children are considered to be in need because of disability, compared with 13% of Caucasians, 9% of Afro-Caribbeans and 7% of those with mixed parentage. If you consider the cultural and language barriers to receiving support as spoken about above, it is understandable that Asian families are less likely to be in receipt of support services and have limited knowledge of direct payment assistance. The research highlights an urgent need for family support and also refutes common myths, such as Asian families being unwilling to receive services such as respite care, or being able to rely on supportive extended family networks (Barn 2006).

Language

There are families who are isolated due to having a child with a disability which is further exacerbated by their first language not being English (see 'Double Discrimination' earlier in this chapter). Many British families go on holiday to a different language speaking country and expect to be spoken to in English. Yes it is known that many people of British origin will not even attempt to try and communicate in another language for fear of making a fool of themselves, or some feel that everyone they meet should speak English. In the UK, however, there is a broad expectation that people whose first language is not English should be able to speak it.

As a professional who will be working with families from diverse backgrounds and cultures, it is good practice to discover how difficult it is to begin to speak another language to native speakers. When we do try to speak a new language to people, we find that they develop respect for us for trying. This respect does not just come from attempting the language, although this is a very good starting point, but from taking time to learn and develop an understanding about a person or family's culture, religion or beliefs, along with the traditions, festivals and celebrations that are important to them.

To make assumptions based on societal or institutionalised influences is not good practice and can be detrimental to how a child and their family are treated, judged and case managed. When working with families from diverse cultures and ethnicities it is important not to make assumptions about their lifestyles, traditions or beliefs. If you do not know whether they observe religious or cultural calendar events, ask them. Some Asian families may only follow part of their traditions while others may be fully devout. Having conversations with families to allow them to tell you where they stand is good practice.

Activity: **Towards adulthood and 'being the same'**

You are working with George, who is is 16 ½. George has muscular dystrophy but does not have any associated learning disabilities and attends a mainstream educational setting. George has said to you that he wants to have a tattoo and try smoking cigarettes. His friends smoke and a few of them have tattoos. He wants to fit in. Although he knows smoking is not good for him, he wants to be able to try it and make a choice about whether he wants to smoke or not. He is very set on having a tattoo of his favourite football club emblem. George's parents are very strict in their beliefs and would not like George's ideas!

What issues would you discuss with George? Can you understand his point of view and how important it is for him to fit in? How would you help George address this with his parents? Consider his rights.

In all the aspects of work and situations you will find when working with children and young people, it is important to look at the situation from their point of view. Think about the situation for George, consider his views and opinions and his need to fit in and make his own choices – you may not agree with his choices but it is important to take the time to consider his perspective.

Taking it further

Barn, R (2006) Improving services to meet the needs of minority ethnic children and families, *Research and Practice Briefings: Children and Families* 13. London: DoH. Available online www.rip.org.uk/resources/publications/frontline-resources/improving-services-to-meet-the-needs-of-minority-ethnic-children-and-families- (accessed 20 November 2015).

Healy, K (2005) *Social Work Theories in Context*. Basingstoke: Palgrave Macmillan.

Sheppard, M (1995) Social Work, Social Science and Practice Wisdom, *British Journal of Social Work* 25(3): 265–293.

Thoburn, T, Chand, A and Procter, J (2005) *Child Welfare Services for Minority Ethnic Families: The Research Reviewed*. London: Jessica Kingsley.

Thompson, N (2006) *Anti-discriminatory Practice*. Basingstoke: Palgrave Macmillan.

Trevithick, P (2006) *Social Work Skills. A Practice Handbook*. Maidenhead: Open University Press.

Chapter 9 | Accessing support and resources

This chapter explores the role of the occupational therapist (OT) and shows how they complement and co-exist with the social work role for children with disabilities. It discusses issues around housing and adaptations and how, with support from an OT, children with disabilities and their families can access a Disabled Facilities Grant (DFG) in order to make their home more accessible for the disabled child. This chapter will look at some universal services that can give support, such as The National Portage Association (Portage) and Children and Family Hubs, and discuss carer's assessments, emergency plans and family group conferences. In addition to this we have given you a list of some resources and websites for you to explore or direct families to for further information. We must add here that we DO NOT endorse or make any recommendations for any of these services: we are just giving information to help you to make your own informed decision. Finally, we briefly discuss a typical process for making a referral to social care.

Occupational therapists

Occupational therapy is the assessment and treatment of physical and psychiatric conditions using specific activities to prevent disability and promote independent function in all aspects of daily life.

Within a children with disability setting you will work closely with OTs. They may be based within a Children with Disability Team, within another team or in a hospital setting and be 'linked' to the team. Each local authority will have their own organisational structures that are slightly different, for example some OTs will be employed by social care and others will be employed by the National Health Service (NHS). In some areas one OT may undertake primary assessments of a child's moving and handling needs within the home environment but also assess and make recommendations for specialist equipment, minor and major adaptations and equipment to support independence and reduce risks to the child and carers.

Let's take a closer look at how an OT working in a Children with Disabilities Team (or perhaps another social care team) might support a young person on your caseload.

Scenario: Helping support Carl

Carl is a child with global developmental delay who is a full-time wheelchair user reliant on carers for all aspects of his day-to-day living. The OT would complete an initial assessment to identify 'meaningful occupations' for Carl. These include the essential activities to meet his care needs and in Carl's case these would be completed by his carers. The OT would look at how best to support and facilitate everyday activities such as eating, sleeping and personal care tasks, assessing for and providing equipment such as postural seating to support feeding, a specialist bed, and a toilet or bathing equipment. The moving and handling involved with accessing each of these would be reviewed and hoists and slings provided if required. If providing the equipment is not enough the OT would assess the home environment as it might need to be altered to ensure all these activities can be promoted; this is where adaptations would be considered and recommended.

We have used the phrase 'meaningful occupations'. The OT assessment is like social work assessments – it is holistic. OTs will also look at other occupations Carl enjoys, either on his own or with family members. It may be that he enjoys interacting with sound and light toys while lying on the floor; the OT will not provide the toys, but they will look at ways of ensuring that Carl can be placed on the floor safely so he can enjoy this play. If he enjoys messy play while sitting, a tray attached to his postural seating provides a surface for this, or the OT will ensure his seating fits under the table so he can get close enough to play. They would look at adaptations to widen a doorway to a family room in order to support Carl spending time with his family. In other words, in addition to the OT looking at essential tasks and ensuring that these can be completed safely and with dignity, they will also look at promoting other activities to ensure that Carl can participate in family life and do things that bring him enjoyment.

Disabled Facilities Grant

If someone living in a property is disabled, they may qualify for a DFG towards the cost of providing adaptations and facilities to enable the disabled person to continue to live there. The legislative framework governing DFGs is provided by the Housing Grants, Construction and Regeneration Act 1996, and the grants are given by local councils under Part I of the Act.

A DFG from the council may allow adaptations or changes to the home, for example to:

» widen doors and install ramps for wheelchair access

» improve/enable access for example to a toilet, bathing, room to sleep and facilities, eg through floor lifts or a downstairs bathroom

A DFG for disabled children under 18 years of age is not means tested but they are only provided following an assessment of need that is undertaken by an OT to identify what is 'necessary' and 'appropriate'. (In certain circumstances, however, some local authorities or councils may decline the request for assistance via a DFG, for example where there has been a payment made following a successful compensation claim, as they will argue that the environmental needs and equipment required for the child would have been factored into the payment.) The current maximum amount available through a DFG in England is £30,000 and in Wales it is £36,000.

To be eligible for a DFG a person in the property must have a permanent and substantial disability and the person applying for the grant (when the DFG is for a child) must:

» own the property or have a secure tenancy

» intend to live in the property following the grant period and the completion of the work (which is currently five years)

A landlord can also apply for a grant for a disabled tenant.

The local authority/district council needs to be happy that the work is:

» necessary and appropriate to meet the disabled person's needs

» 'reasonable and practicable' and can be done depending on the age and condition of the property

The OT will usually oversee and monitor the progress for arrangement of the installation of specialist equipment, also ensuring that facilities' positioning and dimensions are as required to meet the disabled person's needs upon completion of the works.

www.careandrepair-england.org.uk/wp-content/uploads/2014/12/DFG-Good-Practice-Guide-30th-Sept-13.pdf

The local authority may in some circumstances recoup some of the cost of adaptations if homes are sold within 10 years. A 'legal charge' may be placed on a property, for example, if it is sold within a five-year period a percentage of the monies would have to be repaid.

If a child has received a DFG and their property is adapted to meet the child's needs but later on further changes are required or the family choose to move to another property, the family may not be able to have additional adaptations agreed either to their previously adapted property or their new property. Another assessment would have to take place to ensure that the need was valid and explore the reasons why the family moved house. The local council could challenge the decision to move from a suitable property and may decline to adapt another one, unless there are exceptional circumstances. It is important that you discuss individual cases with the OTs and consult legislation and guidance to ensure that you are not giving any incorrect advice to families, particularly as this is not an area of social work specialism: OT colleagues would be the lead professional rather than the social worker. Managing expectations is an important part of the OT role in the area of DFGs and the social worker can support this. At the time of going to print some arrangements for the DFG are undergoing changes and the 'Better Care Fund' is being introduced, so aspects of grant management may change.

Scenario: Arranging a DFG

Shabeena was referred to the Children with Disabilities Occupational Therapy team for an assessment of need in her aunt's property. She had recently been orphaned and her aunt was hoping to provide a home for Shabeena, but she was unsure if this would be feasible given Shabeena's disability and complex needs. While working on this case the OT, Violet, liaised with colleagues in health and social care, including the Looked-After Children social worker, physiotherapists, health OT and wheelchair services. Additionally, Violet was required to work jointly with colleagues from another locality as the aunt's property is in a neighbouring county; responsibility for Shabeena remains with Low Town where Violet works. Violet already knew Shabeena and was therefore familiar with her family history and abilities within her home and school environments, so was well placed to assess her needs and be mindful of the impact of her recent experiences on her well-being. Violet was also able to compare her presentation and mannerisms before and after the loss of her mother and highlight any concerns in relation to how Shabeena was coping.

Upon receiving the referral Shabeena's case was allocated and an initial assessment completed within three weeks. This quick response was essential as information from the assessment was required to ensure that the Looked-After Children's social worker had the relevant information to take to court to support decision making for Shabeena's placement. Violet also had to get the agreement of managers to work outside of the county as home visits were required to ensure that Shabeena's needs were being addressed. The assessment considered the impact

> *of Shabeena and her behaviours on her cousins, who she was now living with, as well as her physical abilities around the home environment, and predicted future long-term access needs. In other words, the assessment was holistic and took into account not only the needs of Shabeena but also of her relatives and how they would manage as a new family unit.*
>
> *Violet recommended an adaptation through a DFG to provide downstairs accommodation for Shabeena. As she was not employed by the local authority who would be providing the adaptation, Violet had to refer Shabeena to her Children with Disability OT colleagues in the relevant county. To reduce repetition Violet shared her assessment with the allocated OT and they conducted a joint visit to the family to discuss who would address specific needs that had been identified in the assessment. Violet was also involved in reviewing the proposed adaptation plans and prescribed necessary equipment, such as specialist postural seating, for Shabeena.*
>
> *The joint working with the OTs in the neighbouring county was very successful. Shabeena settled well in her new home and the equipment provided increased her independence.*

DFG works will only be agreed by the district council after seeing confirming evidence that the property is the disabled person's permanent/long-term residence.

Risk assessments

An OT may carry out risk assessments, for example moving and handling plans to ensure the child is able to transfer or move position safely. When undertaking an assessment of a child with a disability in the home environment, depending upon the complexity of the situation, the OT will often liaise with you as the social worker to ensure that it is a holistic assessment. They would also consult the social worker if there were any concerns about parental capacity, safeguarding concerns about a child's welfare or other issues such as overcrowding or a chaotic home environment. By chaotic we might mean that the parents were not motivated to meet the child's needs because there were lots of things going on in the house, and perhaps the child was not accessing education or had challenging behaviour and the parents were struggling to put boundaries and routines in place. If the family did not already have an allocated social worker, and the OT had any concerns, they should make a referral to the appropriate department for a referral to social care, which might result in an assessment of need for the child by a social worker.

An OT may undertake a risk assessment, for example because a child's bedroom door has a lock on the outside. We talk about locks on doors further in Chapter 2, and look at how an OT and social worker would work together to explore the risks associated with locks on doors. It is important to say here, however, that if you do come across a bedroom door that is being locked this must be explored further with parents and/or carers. A lock on a bedroom door must only be used as a last resort, and all other possible solutions to manage risks should be explored; you should always ensure that you discuss this with your line manager, too.

Safe areas

An OT may undertake a risk assessment if a child is displaying self-injurious behaviour or has a profound disability, and may conclude that there is a need for a 'safe area'.

A safe area, as its name suggests, is 'safe' for children (or adults) who may be unsafe within their normal environment or bed. The safe area is versatile, can be designed specifically for individual special needs, and is often used for children with complex needs such as autism, epilepsy or challenging behaviour. Examples of situations where a safe area might be considered include a child with autism who bangs their head on the wall or floor as they like the sensory feedback, or a child who cannot cope with big spaces so likes to hide and curl up in a small confined area. The safe area may be large enough so the child can stand up or sleep in it, or it may be small and cosy. There are also safe beds with internal padding, or padding can be placed on the internal bedroom walls, depending on the individual's needs and the room that the safe area has to fit into. These safe areas allow the child to relax and chill out and will often be used when their behaviour is starting to escalate or to 'cool down'. When a child is sleeping in the safe area, their parents can have confidence that they cannot hurt themselves, or that the risk is at least reduced. An example of a safe area can be seen at www.safespaces.co.uk/safespaces-films/.

A safe area is something that would not necessarily be funded by a local authority and individual councils may interpret the legislation differently.

Specialist equipment

An OT will undertake assessments to support specific activities to prevent disability and promote independent function in all essential aspects of daily life. This may become more complicated when a child has complex needs that require specialist equipment, however, and the child has respite stays in another environment. The OT may then need to look at what equipment is available in the second environment, especially if the child needs equipment that is not easily transported. Smaller equipment, such as a toilet frame or slings, are more likely to be provided for the second environment, but it is not usually possible to replicate fixed equipment such as a ceiling track hoist as it is not the child's primary residence. The authors are aware of circumstances where OTs have had to support families to approach charities for funding for equipment, for example when there is a shared care arrangement between the divorced parents of a child. DFGs do not fund equipment, so any necessary equipment, including hoists at a second address, would have to be agreed with the local authority or a supportive charity.

An OT may assess that a child needs a specialist bed to give independent access, moving and handling or for health and safety reasons. A child could also require a specialist bed for health reasons, such as needing to angle the mattress base to support posture, or for health tasks, such as managing secretions, respiration and accommodating medical tubes. These beds can also be padded to make safe areas as discussed above. Some beds need to have methods to enclose the bed for the child's safety but also have quick access for an emergency. See: www.bakare.co.uk/solutions/special-needs-beds/. It is essential for the OT to advise carers, in writing, about the safe use of the bed and not using it as a method of restraint.

Attend meetings

You need to think about inviting the OT to meetings that you may be having for a child with a disability, such as Child in Need Meetings, Interim Child Protection Case Conferences (ICPCC), ICPCC reviews, Looked-After Children reviews or Short Breaks reviews. OTs can provide valuable information about the child and the family dynamics as they see the family 'in action' and can give you a different perspective on how a family functions and how routines are working etc. You can also share information with the OT, such as the best way to communicate with the child, and any worries and concerns you may have about the child and their disability or any safeguarding issues. It is very helpful to get feedback from other professionals who work with the families you work with and who get to spend time in their homes.

Children and family hubs

The government put early intervention and prevention at the heart of its recent spending review and as a result, Sure Start Children's Centres are being reshaped as Children and Family Hubs. The aim is to achieve holistic and preventative approaches to early intervention to provide the best outcomes for children, with pooled budgets for local authorities, health and well-being boards and local partners (4Children 2014).

Many Children and Family Hubs are key resources for providing early help intervention, such as:

» Drop-in facilities for support and advice

» Child and family health services, including antenatal support

» Early years education services and play groups (stay and play)

» Speech and language and family learning approaches

» Crèche facilities while parents are attending educational courses on site

» Pre-school for 2–3 year olds

» Support for special educational needs and disabilities

» Adult education and support from Jobcentre Plus

» Parenting courses, such as Triple P, autism awareness or self-esteem

» Father's groups offering them status as an equal partner

» Counselling for children, young people and parents

Many Hubs are also used as contact centres for parents who have supervised contact with their looked-after children. Some centres also offer family support staff who work with families in their own homes to assess their needs and develop individual action plans to address issues that have been identified. They may also help support families with issues such as housing and debt management.

Portage

The National Portage Association provides a home-visiting educational service for pre-school children. They support children with additional needs and help parents to engage with their child in meeting these needs. Portage is currently still a free service. A health visitor could help with referrals to such services although you should also be able to make referrals.

Support from dogs

Hearing dogs for deaf people: this is a registered charity that trains dogs to help deaf people. The dogs alert deaf people to important sounds such as the telephone, doorbell, fire alarms and other danger signals, helping a deaf person to become more independent. They are working dogs and will alert the deaf young person by touching them with their paw or nose in order to gain their attention to what is happening and indicating there is danger. Hearing dogs are provided to the deaf person free of charge (following certain criteria and assessment); the charity match the hearing dog to a specific person and the dog is trained to their individual needs. A hearing dog is a registered 'assistance dog' and the Equality Act 2010 allows them to have access to public places to assist the deaf person in the community. The website for more information is: www.hearingdogs.org.uk.

Guide dogs for the blind: Guide Dogs is a working name of The Guide Dogs for the Blind Association. There is no minimum age for guide dogs for the blind but they tend to start to support young people around their teens. They help promote a visually impaired person to have mobility and freedom, whether blind or partially sighted. They provide trained guide dogs to visually impaired people to allow them to live independently within the community; rehabilitation services to children and adults to become independent with their daily living; and help with long cane mobility training and support communication. Guide Dogs now provide buddy dogs for children and young people with sight loss across the UK. They help give companionship and independence to the child, helping them manage their disability and giving a sense of attachment and responsibility while helping build a child's self-esteem, confidence and communication skills at the same time. Buddy dogs are matched to specific children, and are selected from dogs that have not qualified to be a guide dog. A child with a buddy dog may go on to have a guide dog in the future. Visit their website on www.guidedogs.org.uk.

Dogs for good: previously called Dogs for the Disabled, the charity was registered in 1988. Assistance dogs at Dogs for Good give support, independence, confidence and a best friend to children with a range of disabilities, including autism. A Dogs for Good autism assistance dog gives the parent and child real independence, and provides a safer environment for the child so they feel more secure. The dog wears a special harness that connects it to both parent and child, the parent gives instructions to the dog and the autistic child is encouraged to walk alongside the dog.

An autism assistance dog gives more independence to the autistic child and their parent, while ensuring the child is safe and unable to run off if they become stressed or anxious. The assistance dog is trained to automatically sit should the autistic child attempt to run off. A fully trained autism assistance dog can help change behaviour by:

» Helping to stop/reduce autistic child running off (bolting)

» Helping stop repetitive behaviour

» Establishing routines

» Supporting the autistic child to manage new surroundings.

(www.dogsforgood.org/how-we-help/assistance-dog/autism-assistance-dogs-children/)

Direct payment support

Within this book we have discussed direct payments and how by having a supported account a parent or carer can have someone to help them manage these payments. Here are some managed account providers for direct payments:

The Rowan www.therowan.org/

Care in Finance www.careinfinance.co.uk

Paypacket www.paypacket.co.uk

Penderels Trust www.penderelstrust.org.uk

Ability Finance www.dcil.org.uk

Enable Payroll www.enable-payroll.co.uk

Family fund

The Family Fund is a UK charity that offers discretionary grants to families who are caring for children aged 17 and under (excluding those children in care) who are disabled or have a serious or life-limiting illness. There is a criterion that must be met in order for consideration to be given to applications.

The Family Fund have their own criteria that they use for eligibility, but all children and young people you are applying for must have '*additional complex needs, or have a serious or life-threatening illness*' and '*there must be evidence that the child or young person's additional needs impact on a family's choices and their opportunity to enjoy ordinary life. The degree of planning and support required to meet their needs must also be much greater than that usually required to meet the needs of children and young people*' (www.familyfund.org.uk).

Mencap

Mencap is a charity that supports people with learning difficulties, their families and their carers. They work to challenge oppression and prejudice for people with disabilities and fight to change the laws in favour of those people with disabilities. Mencap offer a host of services such as helping young people gain employment and attend college courses, and offer advice with personal budgets and respite. In addition to this they run residential/day care services and leisure groups that are important to so many people with a learning disability, and their families. A young person who has a personal budget or direct payment could commission the services of a worker from Mencap to manage their personal care or for social inclusion. Mencap also support with advocacy services. See www.mencap.org.uk.

Patient advice liaison service (PALS)

Many parents and carers of children with disabilities and complex health conditions will spend a lot of time at hospital with their child. This can be a frightening and daunting time and unfortunately not always a positive experience. Parents and carers can get a variety of support from PALS at their local hospital. Each hospital should have a PALS and they offer confidential advice, help and information on health-related matters and are a point of contact for families and carers. They can also help resolve concerns or problems and will give information about the NHS complaints procedures. To find a local PALS see www.nhs.uk/chq/pages/1082.aspx.

Carers' assessments

It is very important to consider the needs of the parent and carers of a child with disabilities, and by doing so, you should note that they are entitled to a parent carer's needs assessment in their own right. This assessment can be combined with one for the child, and could be carried out by the same person at the same time; however, in the authors' experience many local authorities have dedicated carers teams that undertake the carer's assessment separately. (We discuss more about carer's assessments in Chapter 1.) A carer's assessment offers the parent/carer an opportunity to discuss what support or services they need to help them in their caring role. The assessment will look at how caring affects different aspects of their life, including physical, mental and emotional needs, and whether they are able or willing to carry on their caring role. It must consider the well-being of the parent/carer and the need to safeguard and promote the welfare of the child cared for, and any other child for whom the parent/carer has parental responsibility (see www.carersuk.org/).

Emergency carer's plan

When families have a crisis, for example if a carer is taken into hospital, it is important that the person they care for (their child with a disability/dependants) is looked after in an emergency. A carer emergency plan (or similar name) can be set up and put in place in order for continuity of care. This plan should provide all relevant, up-to-date information that gives clear instructions about things such as the child's care regime and medications, allergies, how to communicate with the child, and the names and contact details of people the parents would want to be contacted in such an emergency. The parents should ensure they carry a card with them at all times stating they have a 'plan'; the card will have an emergency number that can be called to have the plan activated. In addition, however, carers could consider having some details about what to do in an emergency on a card, and put this in the child's school bag or in a place where it can be easily accessed, perhaps at school on file or on the fridge door – anywhere it can be found quickly in an emergency.

There are services such as Carers UK that will help arrange an emergency plan for a parent/carer and in the authors' experience they have often been discussed following a carer's assessment to ensure that such eventualities are explored. Also see the Local Offer in your area (see www.carersuk.org or put carer's emergency card into the search engine and your local area).

Family group conference (FGC)

FGCs are used for a variety of circumstances and situations, especially when there are concerns about a child's welfare within the child protection arena. This can be essential, particularly to prevent a family breakdown when families reach crisis point and to avoid the child being placed into the care of the local authority. A FGC can identify family members and/or close friends who are able to step in either in an emergency or to prevent emergencies and offer ongoing support. Families, including extended family members, are supported by a FGC coordinator to prepare for the meeting. During the meeting social workers and any other professionals will discuss the concerns, worries and what support they feel would help the family, and raise questions with the family about what support they could offer and make available. The meeting would then allow the family members time (usually on their own) to make their plan, and own it. This allows the family to have control over their own situations rather than having outside agencies becoming involved. It may be necessary to consider how you can arrange for extended family members to receive training if, for example, the child has complex health needs, as this is often a barrier that prevents family members from taking on a caring role. FGCs are an effective way to make safe plans for children, enabling many to stay within their family network as an alternative to going into care, and are cost-effective. Each local authority will have their own policy and procedures about the use of FGCs.

Securing services – resource panel

Once you have completed your Social Care Assessment and identified any unmet needs that require specialist services, it is usual practice that you as the child's allocated social worker will present your case to a panel to request those services. These panels may have different names in different local authorities, and serve different purposes, such as: Resource Allocation Panel (RAP), Complex Needs Panel, Support Panel, Joint Agency Panel or Access to Care Resources Panel. There may be different panels depending upon the type of care packages you are seeking, for example you may go to a RAP, chaired by budget holders at Team Manager level, to request a small package of care such as a direct payment for personal care, and to another panel chaired by Senior Managers (Service Managers etc) to request for a child to be accommodated and become a looked-after child. In order for panels to function they have to be 'quorum' (have a minimum number of members in order to transact business and make decisions legally).

We will look at RAPs. A RAP will approve care packages for specialist services, ie not those that can be met at Universal or Targeted level. The panels are usually made up of professionals from different services, eg a team manager from the social work team, a team manager from fostering and a team manager from a respite unit that offers specialist support to children with disabilities. The RAP may agree, decline or defer a decision for more information. They may also give advice and recommendations for other services that may meet the need, ie at Universal level, or additional services such as a referral to family support or an FGC. The RAP will monitor care packages and may only agree some for a time limited period.

It is usual practice for the allocated social worker to complete a report for the RAP that gives a brief history of the circumstances, the current difficulties and strengths within the family and how the family have tried to meet this need with their own resources. They should identify the unmet need and how the service being requested addresses the gap. They should also state what other services may be in place, such as family support team, CAMHS or a hospice. The social worker will make a request for the service.

Each panel will consider:

> » The social worker's report and Social Care Assessment
>
> » The opinion of specialists that may have been requested (eg CAMHS, paediatrician)
>
> » Other supporting evidence (school reports)
>
> » The child or young person's perspective and the parents' views

The panel may approve packages of care such as:

> » Direct payments – these may be for personal care or short breaks
>
> » Overnight short breaks at specialist respite provision or family foster care
>
> » Other packages of care, eg commissioned services/spot purchase care packages

In the authors' experience parents/carers do not usually attend this type of panel. If a parent/carer or young person was unhappy with the decision or outcome they could appeal in writing or make an official complaint using the local authority's complaints procedure.

If you are completing your Social Care Assessment and identify that a family is in urgent need of support and services, it is normal practice that you do not wait until the completion of your assessment or the next available panel. Instead, you would discuss emergency decisions with the Team Manager (usually the budget holder) to agree that the service be put in place as soon as practicably possible and then the decision would be ratified by the RAP retrospectively.

As discussed above, different panels may agree different things and some of these panels may be multi-agency panels rather than being made up of different services within the same organisation. For example, a panel may comprise professionals, usually senior managers, from health, education and social care. This panel may be known as a Joint Agency Panel and would agree a care package that is jointly funded by each of the three agencies (tri-part); they may not all pay the same percentage.

It is usual practice, in the authors' experience, that when a child is being considered for joint funding they would usually have already been assessed as presenting with severe/exceptional needs, and with clear evidence that mainstream provision could not adequately or sustainably meet the child's assessed needs. Joint Funded Placement will be subject to regular review and based on clear joint planning arrangements.

Whichever panel you are attending and presenting your case to, it is essential that you prepare for this and know your case inside out, as you will be put through your paces by the panel members; some of the recommendations made by a panel can be life-changing for the child (when they are going to become a looked-after child, for example), so it is essential that these processes are rigorous.

Continuing care

The Department of Health 2010 have set out a National Framework for NHS Continuing Healthcare.

A continuing care package will be required when a child or young person has needs arising from disability, accident or illness that cannot be met by existing universal or specialist services alone. The Framework sets out a Decision Support Tool (DST) in relation to enabling immediate decisions on eligibility so that the child's immediate needs can be met. It details principles of assessment whereby the child must be at the very heart of a continuing care assessment process.

There are three key considerations that are paramount in children's continuing care:

» Respecting parents – experts in their child or young person's care and as primary carers.

» The child's home is the centre of caring.

» A child's right to education.

The provision of Continuing Care for children is dependent on the individual meeting the identified eligibility criteria:

» They are under the age of 18 years

» Has complex health needs that include behavioural, emotional, mental health or physical disabilities

» Has identified health needs that cannot be met by existing Universal, Targeted or Specialist local health services, and a checklist indicates the need to progress referral to a full assessment to establish eligibility for Continuing Care

» They have a rapidly deteriorating condition that requires a care package to support end of life care.

To determine the criteria, considerations need to be given to each of the domains below (DH 2010b:para 27:36):

- » Behaviour
- » Psychological and emotional needs
- » Communication
- » Mobility
- » Nutrition
- » Continence
- » Skin and tissue viability
- » Breathing
- » Drug therapies and medication: symptom control
- » Seizures

Each domain is divided into levels describing a hierarchy of need, and given a weighting (not score): no needs, low, moderate, high, severe, priority. Not all domains have the same weighting, based on the principle that some domains reflect health needs more than others.

To look at one of the domains in relation to breathing, you will recall the case scenario of Paul in Chapter 6. His breathing, being identified as severe, would be assessed along with his complex heart condition and the impact this has on his treatment and daily care needs.

In relation to maintaining a child's safety, which is a consideration in most of the domains listed above, here is an example of the criteria that meet a high risk level. A child who requires one-to-one support throughout the day and night from a specifically trained carer to meet their care needs arising from underlying medical conditions, which also requires a high level of risk arising from intense and/or unpredictable care and support, is considered as high risk needs in an assessment. One example to explain this simply could be a child that has a tracheotomy or a central line: they will require care and attention throughout the day and night, which means that parents will require training themselves and also support from trained staff to help them manage.

(www.nhs.uk/CarersDirect/guide/practicalsupport/Documents/National-frame work-for-continuing-care-england.pdf)

Referral to social care

Prior to making any referral to social care it would be our recommendation that you explore universal services, as there are many different types of support available within your local community: we remind you about the Local Offer that each local authority has a duty to provide, which gives details of services and activities on offer for children with SEND (see our Chapter 1 for more information).

If you are reading this chapter from a non-social care perspective and/or you are perhaps working with a child with a disability who does not already have a social worker, and you think that a Social Care Assessment is required, you will have to consider making a referral to social care (or supporting the family to do this themselves). You need to get consent from the family if you are making a referral (unless you have child protection concerns). Each local authority may have slightly different processes for how they receive and allocate their contacts and progress them to a referral, but below is an overview diagram to show what often happens. You need to remember, however, that each Children with Disabilities Team will have their own criteria and not all children will automatically meet the criteria for support from a specialist disability social worker/team, although a parent/carer is entitled to an assessment of need for their disabled child. If a family moves to a new area they may not receive the same service, and different local authorities interpret legislation slightly differently, so the assessments of need may not identify identical unmet needs.

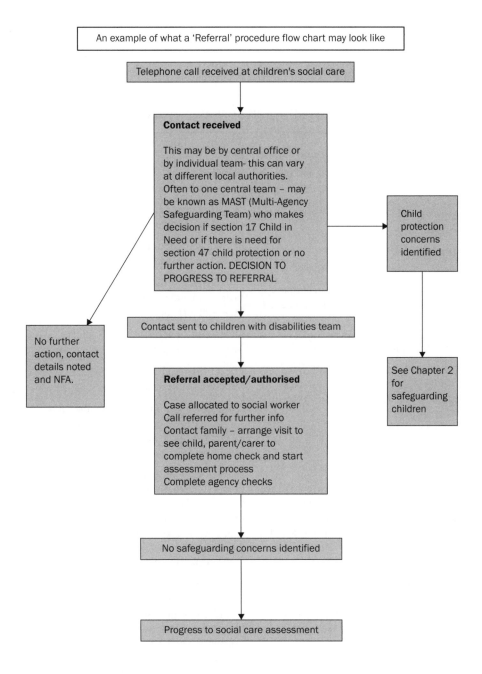

An example of what a 'Referral' procedure flow chart may look like

Telephone call received at children's social care

Contact received

This may be by central office or by individual team- this can vary at different local authorities. Often to one central team – may be known as MAST (Multi-Agency Safeguarding Team) who makes decision if section 17 Child in Need or if there is need for section 47 child protection or no further action. DECISION TO PROGRESS TO REFERRAL

Child protection concerns identified

No further action, contact details noted and NFA.

Contact sent to children with disabilities team

See Chapter 2 for safeguarding children

Referral accepted/authorised

Case allocated to social worker
Call referred for further info
Contact family – arrange visit to see child, parent/carer to complete home check and start assessment process
Complete agency checks

No safeguarding concerns identified

Progress to social care assessment

Taking it further

Here are a few useful websites:

General/miscellaneous support services and resources

MPS Society – The Society for Mucopolysaccharide Diseases is the only UK charity supporting individuals and families affected by MPS, Fabry and related diseases. These are progressive, life-limiting genetic conditions.
www.mpssociety.org.uk

Action for Sick Children
www.actionforsickchildren.org.uk/

SCOPE provide a wide range of support for disabled children and adults and their families.
www.scope.org.uk/support/disabled-people/local/about

Dame Vera Lynn Children's Charity for children under five years old with cerebral palsy (and other motor learning difficulties).
www.dvlcc.org.uk/

Muscular Dystrophy UK
www.musculardystrophyuk.org/

RNID (Royal National Institute for Deaf People) a charity that aims to achieve a better quality of life for those who are deaf or hard of hearing, offering services and information.
www.rnid.org.uk

Communication Matters: A UK charity that supports people who find communication difficult because they have little or no clear speech. For more information visit.
www.communicationmatters.org.uk

National Autistic Society
www.autism.org.uk/

Autism Helpline – www.autism.org.uk/enquiry

Afasic supports parents with children who have difficulties talking and understanding language.
www.afasic.org.uk/

Cystic Fibrosis
www.cysticfibrosis.org.uk/

Down's Syndrome Association (DSA)
www.downs-syndrome.org.uk/

Disabled Living Foundation (DLF) supports independent living:
www.dlf.org.uk

National Deaf Children's Society
www.ndcs.org.uk

Disability Rights UK
www.disabilityrightsuk.org/

SENSE offer support, information and guidance for families and carers supporting a child with a sensory impairment.
www.sense.org.uk

Contact a Family is a national charity for families with disabled children. They offer advice, information and support, help parents get support from one another, and campaign for equal rights. (They also have an A-Z directory of conditions.)
www.cafamily.org.uk

VoiceAbility is a UK charity who work to help support people who are vulnerable and/or marginalised to have their voices heard and respected, offering advocacy services. They also have a training team of 'experts by experience' for disability who are supported by non-disabled colleagues experienced in supporting people with disabilities and mental health difficulties.
www.voiceability.org/

Child Autism UK provides services to enable children to overcome difficulties with communication, learning and life skills, and gives families the techniques and strategies to cope with autism through the use of Applied Behaviour Analysis (ABA). Child Autism UK also provides training and a network for ABA professionals working with young children. They were formerly known as Peach – Parents for the Early Intervention of Children with Autism. www.childautism.org.uk	**The Makaton Charity** www.makaton.org

Carer and sibling support websites

Special Needs Jungle helps parents get support for the statementing process and sifting through the jungle of SEN information. www.specialneedsjungle.com **The Princess Royal Trust for Carers** provides information, guidance and support. www.carers.org **Face2Face** Parents supporting parents of disabled children. www.scope.org.uk/support/services/befriending/about-face-2-face **SIBS** is a UK charity for people who grow up with a brother or sister who have any disability, long-term chronic illness or life-limiting condition. An excellent site with all sorts of information. www.sibs.org.uk/	**Carers Direct** is an information resource providing advice and support for carers. www.nhs.uk/Carersdirect **Parents of Disabled Children** An online support forum for parents and carers of disabled children. www.parentsofdisabledchildren.co.uk **Support for fathers** of disabled children can be found at the Fatherhood Institute's website. www.fatherhoodinstitute **Young Carers** A website for young carers, including siblings, with excellent support and information sections such as 'How I feel' and 'Who can help me?' with interactive videos. www.youngcarers.net

Palliative care/end of life support

National Council for Palliative Care www.ncpc.org.uk **Dying Matters Coalition** www.dyingmatters.org **Good Life, Good Death, Good Grief** www.goodlifedeathgrief.org.uk	**The National Association of Funeral Directors** www.nafd.org.uk **The Natural Death Centre** www.naturaldeath.org.uk

Together for Short Lives www.togetherforshortlives.org.uk/ There are many hospices across the UK for children and families so we are not able to list them all. We found one of the best websites for finding a children's hospice in your local area was **ehospice** – they give advice and support for patients, employees and families of patients, and up-to-date news, changes and research for palliative and hospice care. The site offers worldwide information but allows you to list all hospices (in their catalogue) in the UK for children (and adults). It listed 67 children's hospices across the UK, giving addresses, telephone and email addresses and website links. www.ehospice.com/uk/en-gb/home.aspx	Child Bereavement Charity www.childbereavement.org.uk **Hospice UK** supports the development of hospice care in the UK and internationally (linked to ehospice). They champion the voice of hospice care and clinical excellence. They help hospice care providers to deliver the highest quality of care to people with life-limiting or terminal conditions and their families. www.hospiceuk.org/about-hospice-care/work-in-hospice-care

Activities

Here are some providers of activities and organised sport and recreational opportunities for people with disabilities at both local and international levels:

British Wheelchair Sports Foundation www.wheelpower.org.uk/WPower/ English Federation of Disability Sports www.efds.co.uk/ Riding for the Disabled Association Incorporating Carriage Driving RDA has nearly 500 groups across the UK who organise activities for a big community of 28,000 riders and carriage drivers). www.rda.org.uk	British Paralympic Association www.paralympics.org.uk/ Great British Wheelchair Basketball Association www.gbwba.org.uk/gbwba/welcome.htm Disability Sports Events www.disabilitysport.org.uk/ Get Kids Going www.getkidsgoing.com/

Further reading

College of Occupational Therapy/British Association of Occupational Therapy www.cot.org.uk.

H M Government Disabled facilities grants www.gov.uk/disabled-facilities-grants/eligibility.

Government Legislation Housing grants, Construction and Regeneration Act 1996 and www. opsi.gov.uk/acts/acts1996/Ukpga_19960053_en_1.

Play Matters (2007) *Toy Libraries: Their Benefits for Children, Families and Communities.* London: National Association of Toy and Leisure Libraries. Available online www.ncb.org. uk/media/195173/capacityreportjune07.pdf (accessed 22 March 2016).

This chapter includes actual thoughts, views and experiences of children and their families on the receiving end of Children's Social Care involvement. It explores disability from the family's perspective and details some of the real-life experiences they have faced. This perspective gives an insight into the attributes of positive social work that makes a difference, with helpful pointers around do's and don'ts when working with families. A special poem has been included, which we feel is inspirational in bringing together the context of this chapter through thought-provoking words of experience.

We would like to take this opportunity to thank each and every one of the young people, parents, carers and siblings who took part in our interviews and gave their valuable and precious time to help inform our practice as social workers, and who shared their stories and experiences with us.

How the information was collated

A questionnaire was designed inviting people to reflect on their own experiences, to identify how they initially felt about having social care intervention and support and to identify what worked well and what actually helped with their situations. Face-to-face interviews and discussions were also undertaken.

The family perspective

1. **We understand how difficult it is as a parent to have to keep sharing information with professionals about your child, especially relating to their disability or complex health needs. What do you feel would help with this?**

"A booklet that has information about the child, that has been filled in by the child, the child's parent(s) and professionals. Information should include their needs, abilities, inabilities, likes, dislikes, strengths, obsessions, triggers etc (similar to person-centred care). The booklet needs to be changeable as the child's needs/preferences may change. This should be carried by the parent(s) so it can be handed to the professional when needed."

"If there was the ability to centralise a computer system that is accessible or compatible to enable social workers and other professionals to look at information that is recorded re health CAMHS."

"If the social worker could have accessed the health system they would have seen the medication and know how this made the child's skin bruise easily, instead of accusing and questioning."

"Health and social working more in partnership together to make communication smoother."

"Too many changes of social worker in a short time, each one wanting to ask for information and background rather than reading it, having to go through story over and over."

"To know how to build trust, social worker should follow the child through the processes."

"Need smoother transition from child to adult as information does not get passed or shared."

"The support for adults drops tremendously."

"There should be a need for social workers to be able to read notes of health and for health professionals to be able to read social care records, as information can be missed when concerns are recorded in separate systems but not always shared."

"There should be one compatible chronology that all professionals can add to as they work or are involved with a child."

"Not everyone turns up at meetings and so information is not shared fully."

"A joint working policy/communication strategy between agencies which enables the information to be shared with relevant professionals, so that families do not have to tell their story more than once."

"Online log, diaries, detailed portfolio."

"It's really frustrating and quite depressing to have to keep telling your story to different people. I feel that there should be some kind of single process that is accepted by all agencies, I remember years ago my children had an early years pack from Portage with a progress folder that had photos and things they had done and achieved in a box; however no one at meetings ever wanted to look at the folder and I carried it about with me, so it did not work across the board but I thought it was a good idea."

"There should be just one report written that explains all the areas such as education, health, learning and sensory needs and this should be accessible to all the professionals involved. It does not matter who leads this but there needs to be a key person who pulls all the information together."

"The Education, Health and Care Plan is designed to cover education, health and social care needs but in practice it is not working as sometimes at meetings one of the areas' representatives do not attend and so not all the areas can be covered together; perhaps this is due to resources."

"It would be better if a co-ordinator collected and passed on the information to other professionals prior to meetings with parents and children."

"If the health professionals make the referral, then a set of notes (background) should be passed on so the social worker can be informed of the disabilities/condition prior to the meeting."

"It is frustrating having to tell your story... but I would rather people ask me things that they don't know: it's better to ask and be honest if you don't know something about my child as not everybody will know everything. It doesn't really bother me now having to tell my story – I'm used to it because we get so many different workers as they are always coming in and out of their jobs."

2. Having had to have social workers involved in your life, could you recall how this felt for you initially when the social worker first visited?

"Fear, worry, upset, anger, inadequacy. People do not always understand that social services are there to help. People automatically relate social workers with having their children removed from their care."

"Our initial visit left us feeling awful even though we knew we hadn't done anything wrong; it made us feel very bad. The social worker approached with aggression and visited with her manager to make it worse, with double questioning, and made us feel guilty."

"Initially it was not a good experience as there had been a report made by school as they were not good at understanding disability related needs and behaviours and were a mainstream school. This resulted in a social worker making an investigation which made us feel initially that we were being accused of hurting our child. However, the investigation resulted in an assessment which identified that there were no concerns but also identified there was a need for support, recognising our child as a child in need which enabled us to access services and support for us and our child. The social worker had been experienced enough to see beyond the panic, and they could see the positives that we had in place for our child."

"There was an initial element of apprehension and anxiety around the expectations of the professional."

"Like they were judging my parenting, taking my children away for respite."

"Initially I had received a telephone call from a social worker saying that due to a change in their systems and requirements, I needed to have a social worker involved in order to continue to receive the support of a couple of hours a week I had already been receiving. I was told I needed to have police checks done on all the family and also that my home would be inspected. This felt awful and was very intrusive and did not make a good start to social work involvement. A trainee social worker had made the call and was unable to answer my questions about why this was happening, and the social worker had been told to make these calls to those who were receiving the service. I didn't feel this was handled well, and we were told that this new system was needed as part of the condition of having a service and if we did not want the involvement we would not get the service any more. We did not want to go through more assessment and it made a negative start. However, when the social worker came to visit she was really good and took the stress out of the process."

"The title 'social worker' conjures up a negative feeling as if you're not doing your job properly as a parent. The social worker needs to aim to dispel these feelings at the onset."

"I was horrified – I only felt that social workers went to 'troubled families' and I felt stigmatised: my own mother said to me "You are the first person in this family to have a social worker." I was perturbed by this from my mother and her perception of us."

3. **As our book aims to promote active social work with children with disabilities, is there anything you can share about how an initial visit from a social worker visiting you and your child could be a positive start to a working relationship with your family?**

"Reassurance; tell them that you are there to help and not judge. Allow the parent(s) to decide whether the first meeting is made within the home or elsewhere. Keep the first meeting informal. Let the parent(s) know that you trust and believe in them and the work they are doing with their child... trust and belief go a long way with struggling parent(s)."

"To be less confrontational."

"Social worker needs to have experience and be able to approach difficult conversations in a respectful and non-judgmental manner."

"The social worker needs to be calm and have a more friendly approach. The social worker should explain they want the best for the child and want to help. Social workers should listen to both parents and the child and listen to views separately and talk to the child on their own and at school. Social worker should be open and honest themselves and tell us in a plain clear way what their concerns are."

"Social workers getting challenged when they have assessed a need that needs a funded resource, which undermines their professional assessment."

"Social workers need to ensure that they have an overview of the family situation beforehand. An initial visit could serve to develop and foster that level of trust required to work in partnership with the family and child/young person."

"Feel like someone is on your side listening to how life really is at home."

"What would be really good is at the first meeting the social worker explains their role and how they can help. To make the first visit as a more 'meet and greet' without an agenda and to talk about how services can support and to ask me what services can support me."

"The social worker needs to be very friendly and approachable and initially promote how a social worker can help the family, giving examples of case studies for example."

"Not so much about the initial visit but when I have had a social worker I found that they didn't visit a lot – it was hit and miss. I didn't get a lot of input from them due to staffing – but I don't want a lot because I know they are there but when I have phoned them when I was in a crisis I didn't get any help because I'm seen as a parent who can cope."

4. **Did the assessment/reports reflect your child and your family's situation? Did it give a true picture or were there bits missing or misinterpreted? Can you give one bit of advice on how an assessment should read?**

"The reports we had were a fair reflection which also showed how our child had changed in his behaviour and regression."

"Assessments sometimes are too long with too many pages, and have a lot of jargon which is not parent friendly. We need more succinct reports written in plain language."

"The first assessment, I did not get a copy, when I got the assessment it did not explain why the assessment was made or what the concerns were. However, the last assessment I had in relation to the disability was a more open and honest report."

"Child in need reports are good as it shows actions needed by everyone and things get followed up, outstanding issues remain on for next time and new issues or needs are added. They are easy to understand and follow my child's progress."

"It is easier when reports are written in plain English."

"The assessments need to be less of a tick box exercise and reveal more of a holistic approach. Perhaps reviewing and developing an assessment tool with children, young people and their families would give a more accurate reflection of what is required."

"Clear and understood which it was."

"The social worker made a really good report with lots of positives and strengths and gave some good examples of what the children had done. Just reading it, if you did not know us, it gives a really good feel for our story."

"The initial one was good and since then it's been hit and miss. They have been thorough but also it's upsetting when you read things in black and white about you and your child and family. I think that when social workers write them they don't always consider how it is for us as parents to read them."

"It must be open and honest and well written, and PROOF-READ and appropriate language used. I don't like it when they say my child is "wheelchair bound"... it is better to say he is a "wheelchair user" and it is better to say a child with a disability not a disabled child. They should ask the parent what language they like (within reason)."

5. **Without disclosing any sensitive and detailed information about you or your child, could you describe some main barriers or difficulties that you found in having a social worker supporting you, your child or your family?**

"Being told what I should or shouldn't do in regards to raising my child. Both me and my child not being listened to. It is my belief that I am the true expert on my child as I am with him more than anyone, I know exactly whom he is and all about him. Reassurance and advice can be helpful though."

"When we needed help with strategies, we were advised to shut our child in a room with no furniture, or ring the out of hours team or to ring the police. He was having outbursts and we needed strategies to help stop and more importantly to prevent the outbursts happening, but initially we had no one who could advise or guide us in a practical way which is what we needed."

"It's a bit of a mine field, no one tells you what to do when you get the diagnosis – you just go out into the world and find your way the hard way."

"We managed for nine years and did not know what support might be out there to help and we found this out a year ago and now we get some support, no one tells you what's out there you seem to stumble across services and people who know things."

"Initially we had two social workers visit when there was a concern to be investigated, they acted as 'bad cop and good cop', one was really nice and the other one was more blunt, but they were both still approachable."

"I cannot think of any barriers; I am able to talk to the social worker openly and I have had a good experience with this involvement."

"I have no perceived barriers and have always seen service intervention, if required, as a positive experience."

"Felt I was being watched/judged."

"The barrier as I see it is the 'system'. The initial phone call we had, which was horrible, was a social worker having to follow instructions from the system and the system causing the changes and the stresses that relate to the changes."

"A social worker saying they need to visit within seven days due to the system that requires them to make visits within a certain timescale; this does not fit sometimes when family have holiday periods or times that these visits are not compatible to the already full timetabled lives. I understand that the children need visiting but the pressure I feel from the social worker saying they have to visit because they are due to visit, rather than visiting because they care and would like to meet with the children, is not in my opinion good family working."

"Due to the system making the changes and telling families they can no longer have a service if they do not have a social worker involved places a danger of some families refusing the involvement, which could result in the respite or support not being there to support the families, which could increase the stresses within the families, and also there could be a risk that with the service no longer going in the child and their family could become more isolated."

"Paperwork and actual appointments can become a barrier as the amount of time that parents are expected not only to attend health appointments with the child, which may include physio and other routine treatments and check ups, and education appointments, there are all the other meetings that we need to attend for social care and also to be available for visits when are lives are already full."

"It would be upsetting to expect certain help and to be offered something different which you deem inappropriate, but the authorities/panel thought otherwise. It would make all the initial meetings a waste of time from the parent's point of view."

"I don't get much support from the social worker. They phoned last summer; I fell and broke both my feet and it took them five days to ring and ask me how I was and I didn't get any support at all. I didn't say I want this and that and the other and therefore I got nothing and my husband had to take six weeks off work to care for me and my child. My husband would not take us both out as we both had wheelchairs. They don't ring us now and we don't get any support, I don't think it will happen now. Some families have some good relationships and their workers sit and listen."

"We are seriously lacking support for siblings. Young Carers Team worker came and said to my other child (who does not have a disability) do you want to go out and climb trees? My child was horrified and wouldn't talk to them again. He didn't want to go out he just wanted things explaining to him, but not all the time. He has seen a lot of things, he has seen his brother fighting for his

life in intensive care at the hospital and needs to talk things through, not going out with other people he did not know, he would be horrified. The 1:1 support at the hospice was great. The social workers should just offer to talk to siblings for an hour or so occasionally."

6. **Do you have any examples of actions or practice from your social worker that stood out as really positive? Whether it was words, advice, guidance or support that other social workers might take as a guide for their practice.**

"Being reassured that I'm doing a really good job. Praise for the work we do as parent(s) of children with needs. Being shown that there is help, and what help is available to me without it being forced onto me. Being shown that there is nothing wrong in asking for or needing a little help, we are only human."

"We now have a social worker who gets down on the floor to his level and talks to him about the things he likes. The social worker listens as he is now finding activities of interest and encouraging our child to partake and enjoy things, for example he is going to have a DJ session to mix some music which is what he likes doing."

"A social worker who is not afraid to get down and play games with our child, and interact with them fully."

"The social worker has been there to support and they have been flexible and available."

"Generally being kind and human."

"A good communicator, finding new ways of keeping in touch such as texting which works well for my work commitments as I cannot always take a call."

"Supported me and my son when I needed her, ie hospital, school, CAMHS and college."

"The social worker we had was very knowledgeable and just had a really good knowledge of services in the area and also had lots of ideas to share around things to try around different strategies. She really knew her stuff."

"Really listening, our social worker had picked up some really key points in the assessment but when assessing she was just having conversations with us but was really listening out for the key points which was really good and skillful."

"The social worker interacted with my children, she spent a lot of time talking and playing with them about their favourite things, she was able to soon get to know them and know how they communicated."

"A friendly face with lots of smiles. Good listening and communication skills."

"One worker took notice of the likes and dislikes of my young person and remembered things – they didn't try and fob me off, and were open and honest that they did not know a lot. I couldn't think of anything else positive about the others."

7. **If you could offer one meaningful quote to reflect what quality is needed to be a good social worker working with children with disabilities, what would you say?**

"It's not a 'mistake', it's an adventure where a lesson was learned."

"A diagnosis is not a label, it's an explanation."

"The biggest disability anyone can have is ignorance."

"A good social worker should always listen to parents as most of us know best."

"Listen."

"My child says that people don't listen to him as they want to ask questions through me most of the time; he wants to be able to give his own views and be asked his own questions."

"Keep the child involved in every step."

"Listen to the parent and the child."

"Social workers working with children/young people with disabilities need to ensure they have the expertise and life experience required to support families who are often experiencing a high degree of stress and conflict in their daily lives. They need patience, compassion and an insight into the impact of the families' caring role."

"To understand a child with a disability and to understand parents' needs."

"Social workers need to try and walk a mile in parents' shoes."

"Social workers need to try and put themselves in a child or young person's shoes to help understand their world and how it looks from their view."

"Be genuinely interested in people's lives and situations."

"To have a genuine interest and to show enthusiasm and have a positive approach."

"If someone says they are going to do something – do it."

"Follow things through and ring up and say if you haven't been able to do it – DON'T FOB ME OFF."

"If I'm not eligible for something, say 'You are not eligible.'"

8. **Did you feel that the social worker really understood what you were experiencing and what life was (or still is) like for you as a parent or carer of a child or young person with a disability? Can you give any examples of why you feel this way?**

"I think they do."

"It is the systems they have to follow that makes it less personal, especially when boxes need to be ticked to meet criteria questions; a form does not always allow real needs and impact to be seen and understood."

"I didn't feel this was the case; there was little life experience and an inability to recognise the impact of caring for and supporting a child/young person with severe learning disabilities. The Adult Care social worker was much more empathetic."

"Listens to me and understands me as a mother and wants the best there can be for my son."

"I had a social worker on a previous occasion ask my daughter if she can stand when she couldn't. The notes should be read before a visit."

"NO – my worker hasn't got a clue!! He doesn't understand the day-to-day difficulties. Parents come to terms with things at different times and in different ways – he does talk to my husband when he is here with me but he hasn't spoken to him or seen him on his own."

9. Any other comments you would like to share which you feel would inform social work practice in this field?

"It's difficult for anyone to truly understand what life is like with a child with health needs as every child is different and therefore each parent goes through different experiences."

"Over time, I've learnt strategies for dealing with and coping with my son's needs. These strategies help all of my family and not just me and my son. Having advice and suggestions for other strategies were helpful, being told what I should/shouldn't be doing wasn't."

"We are lucky as our social worker really understands us and knows it is not easy for our child or us at times and shows this in the way he cares and tries to support and share ideas, strategies and to find new activities for our child to join in with."

"I believe, like teachers, social workers working with children/young people with disabilities, should have to undergo a level of special needs and disabilities training as part of their training programme."

"Young people do want professionals working with them, encouraging late teens to go into the profession would be ideal."

"Transition is a worry – I asked about transition for my child. "Set something up yourself" was the response. When I asked what post-19 care is there? There is nothing. I was told to set it up – it's scary: you should consider what type of worry that is for us, it really is, there are no services."

"I believe the relationship you have with your social worker makes the difference to the support you get."

"Read the minutes of meetings and put in them what was said and read them."

"Check minutes of the meetings with family members – ring us and check with the parent if you are unsure. Send a letter with them (or email) asking us to let you know if they are not correct before you send them out to everyone else – you presume they are OK and they may not be and that is the information that feeds into other assessments."

"Not all disabled children sleep, some do not because of their condition. Consider sleep deprivation and how families are not functioning well and how this affects people differently. Sleep or not having sleep can change families."

"Respite – gives us a break, it means we don't have to give him his feeds for that day/night or get them ready and we don't have to have eyes in the back of our head for one night."

"Medication is not always the answer."

Children and young people's voice

Advocating is speaking out on behalf of children and young people who do not have a voice to express their needs, views and wishes. It is good to sometimes try to step into a child's shoes and imagine what they would be saying about themselves, their needs or their situation if they were able to. It helps to keep your practice and approach child focused and to be mindful of their situation. Based on the authors' experience of working with children, including babies, and young people with varying levels of disabilities here are a few quotes written by us that we felt the children we knew would be sharing and expressing. The views of some of the children who we did speak to within our research have also been included with these comments.

"I need you to speak on my behalf, learn my signs and body language, look closely at my movements – they are all I have to communicate with."

"I need you to take plenty of time when getting to know me and in communicating with me, be patient, watch and wait for my responses: they may not be verbal."

"Please treat me with respect and dignity, don't talk past me or about me when I am there; keep me involved as much as you can."

"I rely on you and others to keep me healthy, I cannot tell you if I am in pain – you need to watch closely and remind others involved to do this too."

"If I have a bad toothache I cannot tell you, it will hurt bad and I may try to do different things to let you know like not eating or drinking."

"I can fully understand you and what you are asking me, but my brain won't allow my mouth to say out the words very quickly or clearly; please be patient and let me try and answer before you finish and asked the next question."

"I can only hear and think about the first two words you say to me – the rest is just a fuzz."

"I will rock back and forth when I am worried: this is my sign that I am not coping in a situation."

"I will put my hands on my ears and will make humming sounds to block out the noises that are too much for me to cope with; this usually happens when my family are all talking and the TV is on."

"I am only a baby so pick me up and interact with me – you will learn more about how I am."

"Don't just talk down at me, get on the floor and play with me – it will help me to see and get to know you."

"I wanted a male keyworker, and currently have one – that's great. I told him I want to do practical activities in a setting that is not like a school. He sorted things for me so I will be going to two places soon and I can go to activities and practical things, like a college. I enjoy having the opportunity to talk alone with my social worker without having my parents to assist me. I was listened to."

Some perspectives from other sources

There are research reports and information from parent surveys that have gathered information from a parent or family perspective on their experience of social work involvement. The information is vast, however we wanted to pull through some of the common themes. There were many parents who felt they had been treated with respect from the social worker, which reflected a positive working relationship between the social workers and the families they worked with. A positive level of parents felt the social worker listened well and was child focused. The survey information also showed positive strengths in parents' understanding of what the social worker is trying to achieve, and also in how they felt about whether the social worker was making a positive difference in their child's life. Parents had shared some general views around their involvement and working relationship with a social worker for their child with a disability, and here is a general summary of views we feel are relevant to this chapter.

"We found having Children's Services involved has been a lifesaver."

"The social worker helped to improve the quality of my child's life and I want to say 'Thank you.'"

"The social worker has communicated well and shown empathy and understanding and has been proactive."

"There needs to be more activities available for children with special needs."

"The social worker has been in tune with my child's needs and also with my family's needs and has been very supportive."

"It is difficult when there is no continuity of staff – although it is understood this cannot be helped, it is difficult to have to get to know a new social worker and their style."

"There needs to be better communication between different agencies."

"The social worker is calm, understanding and a good communicator, and has been very professional with a caring side when needed."

"The social worker made the transition for our child into adult service smooth by getting the adult social involved early and co-worked through the transition."

'Welcome to Holland'

As you may recall, in the introduction of this book we included a poem, 'Welcome to Holland', written by Emily Perl Kingsley; her words of honesty, experience and the wonderful analogy help to explain how it feels when your life plan is changed and you have to learn acceptance and to adapt to a new life. Well, Emily Perl Kingsley wrote an equally warming part two to her analogical poem, one that finds us further along the journey of life-changing experiences and the acceptance we do eventually find.

As this chapter has explored views and experiences from the family perspective we thought it fitting to end with these wonderful and thought-provoking words of wisdom from a person who has taken their journey and been able to see the positives and rewards in her changed life. Luckily she wrote and shared her thoughts and we thank her for this. See what you think!

'Welcome to Holland' (Part 2)

I have been in Holland for over a decade now. It has become home. I have had time to catch my breath, to settle and adjust, to accept something different than I'd planned.

I reflect back on those years past when I had first landed in Holland. I remember clearly my shock, my fear, my anger – the pain and uncertainty. In those first few years, I tried to get back to Italy as planned, but Holland was where I was to stay. Today, I can say how far I have come on this unexpected journey. I have learned so much more. But, this too has been a journey of time.

I worked hard. I bought new guidebooks. I learned a new language and I slowly found my way around this new land. I have met others whose plans had changed like mine, and who could share my experience. We supported one another and some have become very special friends.

Some of these fellow travellers had been in Holland longer than I and were seasoned guides, assisting me along the way. Many have encouraged me. Many have taught me to open my eyes to the wonder and gifts to behold in this new land. I have discovered a community of caring. Holland wasn't so bad.

I think that Holland is used to wayward travellers like me and grew to become a land of hospitality, reaching out to welcome, to assist and to support newcomers like me in this new land. Over the years, I've wondered what life would have been like if I'd landed in Italy as planned. Would life have been easier? Would it have been as rewarding? Would I have learned some of the important lessons I hold today?

Sure, this journey has been more challenging and at times I would (and still do) stomp my feet and cry out in frustration and protest. And, yes, Holland is slower paced than Italy and less flashy than Italy, but this too has been an unexpected gift. I have learned to slow down in ways too and look closer at things, with a new appreciation for the remarkable beauty of Holland with its tulips, windmills and Rembrandts.

I have come to love Holland and call it Home. I have become a world traveller and discovered that it doesn't matter where you land. What's more important is what you make of your journey and how you see and enjoy the very special, the very lovely, things that Holland, or any land, has to offer. Yes, over a decade ago I landed in a place I hadn't planned. Yet I am thankful, for this destination has been richer than I could have imagined!

Emily Perl Kingsley

Reproduced with our acknowledgement, respect and gratitude – Julie Adams and Diana Leshone.

This chapter gives a variety of case scenarios and activities, in addition to those within each chapter, that can be completed by the social worker and Practice Educators and their students on placement or within supervision and/or team meetings to support Continued Professional Development (CPD). The exercises are also suitable for those social workers undertaking training on their Assessed and Supported Year in Employment (ASYE) and they evidence their learning and reflective practice on each activity. After this chapter we have included a useful glossary of some of the terms, acronyms and disabilities you may come across when working with children with disabilities.

We have tried to keep the exercises related to the chapters in the book, but you will also recognise the relevance in some other chapters.

Chapter 1: Legislative frameworks for supporting children with disabilities

Case scenarios: Assessing

Scenario 1: Differing perspectives

The police report that they were called out to the family home following a report of shouting and swearing. On attending the property, the door was opened by a 15-year-old boy, Alex. Police submitted a report to Children's Social Care stating that the condition of the property was extremely poor. Police described that the kitchen was overflowing with dirty pots and pans, dirty laundry stacked in the hallway, minimal furniture and bedding and the bed sheets appeared very tatty. Following this information, Children's Social Care visited the property and did not make the same observations; they stated that conditions were found to be acceptable and the bedding was seen to be 'acceptable'. The house was not too warm but was not really cold. Alex said he was OK and he was doing some homework. His sister Susan, who has a gastrostomy tube and carers who call at the home twice a day to support with personal care, was at home and smiled at the workers.

What might this indicate about the both Alex's and Susan's care, and what impact might this have upon them? Are you worried? If so why, if not why not?

Scenario 2: Having too much fun?

Henry has Down's syndrome and he is undergoing tests at school to assess him for an attachment disorder. He is 11 years old. Henry really loves to go to the youth club every Tuesday; he never misses and really enjoyed the evening tonight playing table tennis because he won the tournament. Tonight Henry seems reluctant to go home at the end of the session. He hasn't given any specific reasons as to why he doesn't want to go home.

What factors might you consider? Are you worried? If so why, if not why not?

Chapter 2: Exploring processes in practice

Safeguarding children quiz

» What type of meeting (can be a discussion) is held when you need to decide if you are going to undertake a child protection investigation because you believe a child may be suffering, or is at risk of suffering, significant harm?

» What type of meeting is held to decide if a child should be made subject to a Child Protection Plan?

» Name six types of professional you might invite to a Child in Need Meeting or a Core Group Meeting, such as a health visitor (this is not one we want you to find).

» Name the four categories of abuse/harm that you must consider when you have decided a child is to be made subject to a Child Protection Plan.

» What type of skill is essential for a social worker in order for them to be able to ascertain the child's voice?

» How many days after a Child Protection Case Conference would you hold your first Core Group Meeting?

» What type of harm is a child deemed to be at risk of when you are considering child protection procedures?

» What type of meeting do you hold when a child is subject to a CPP?

» How many days after your Strategy Meeting would you hold a Child Protection Case Conference?

» What is the key legislation that underpins your social work practice?

William

In Chapter 2 we discussed Olivia and William when we considered whether it was acceptable (as a last resort) to use a lock on Olivia's bedroom door, or in William's case it was a lock on a tent, in his bedroom, that his parents were using as a restraint to keep William safe. We asked the question 'to lock' or 'not to lock'. Please see Olivia's Child in Need Plan below: it was completed at the end of her Social Care Assessment and high-lights what needs to happen to help keep Olivia safe, and what the professionals need to do and consider in order to ensure Olivia is kept safe and by when. Following the CIN Meeting steps were then taken to assess the risks around Olivia having the lock on her door. A meeting took place that looked at Olivia's 'Risk to Safety Assessment Agreement' being drawn up, which will then continue to be reviewed at her CIN meetings.

Now you have looked at Olivia's CIN Plan and have an idea of what goes into a plan and what one may look like, we would like you to write a Plan for William. We would just like to say that each local authority will have their own ideas of what a CIN Plan should look like and what it should include and will most likely have their own templates, but we have put one together that we hope is on the same lines as those you may use elsewhere. Please go back to Chapter 2 and read William's scenario again, consider the main issues in the story and then read 'Intervention and support offered to William and his family', below. Put these issues, and any others you can think of, into the plan.

Intervention and support offered to William and his family

» *Social Care Assessment was completed and regular Child in Need visits and reviews held.*

» *Advice provided in respect of safety at night and not locking the tent, a written agreement and risk assessment formulated to ensure that William is not being locked in a tent at night time and with appropriate strategies for parents.*

» *Family Support became involved, offering assistance with strategies to help manage both children's behaviours.*

» *Liaison with school for arranging William's Education, Health and Care Plan to support with transition to specialist educational setting.*

» *Family Group Conference to explore help available from any extended family and friends.*

» *Direct Payments provided for a short break for six hours a week to take William out and give parents a break.*

» *Direct Payments agreed for Friendly Carers who provide one hour of personal care support a week during term time and ten hours in school holidays.*

Child's name: Olivia Green	Social worker: Jenni Jinks	Date of plan: 10-02-16

Main issues and aim of plan for child:

Olivia is a young girl whose behaviour at times can be very challenging. Olivia has a diagnosis of autism spectrum disorder and ADHD. Due to Olivia's disability/diagnosis, she requires supervision at all times. She has no sense of danger, for example Olivia will attempt to light the oven, flood the sink, drink disinfectant and run off into the road. The assessment also identified that Olivia is being locked in her bedroom at night. Mr and Mrs Green are Olivia's main carers and they are finding the constant supervision and management of Olivia difficult, so they have requested respite and support to be able to continue to care for Olivia. There are many things that are positive, such as Olivia is well cared for and loved; Mr and Mrs Green feel that they work well together; Olivia is provided with lots of praise when she is displaying behaviours which are encouraged; Olivia is being supported by a number of professionals; and she enjoys school.

The aim of the plan is for Olivia to remain in the care of Mr and Mrs Green and for them to feel that they are supported to enable this to continue, and for all professionals to work together with Olivia, Mr and Mrs Green and each other to ensure that Olivia is able to thrive and achieve the best of her ability.

Who is responsible for the change?	What is causing us to be concerned?/What action do we need to take?	By when?	How will we recognise the actions have been completed? State goals for individuals and/or organisation concerned.
Jenni Jinks	Mr and Mrs Green are worried that they will be unable to continue to care for Olivia without a break. They have highlighted the need for respite care. Jenni needs to complete the panel application to request respite for Olivia at the Happy Days respite centre and request Direct Payments be put in place.	Next Child in Need (CIN) meeting.	Jenni would have completed a panel application and a decision will have been made. Mr and Mrs Green will be receiving a break from their caring role, which will enable them to be able to continue to care for Olivia.
Eric Helper (CAMHS) Dr Fixer (paediatrician)	Olivia's behaviour is very challenging at the moment and parents and professionals are worried about the impact this could be having on Olivia. Olivia's medication needs to be reviewed so that she is taking medication to help her feel calm.	Next CIN meeting.	Olivia will be taking medication. Olivia will be feeling much calmer and behaving better.
Irene Learner (School)	Olivia responds well to sensory play/activities, therefore it has been highlighted that this needs to be increased within the different environments, especially school.	Ongoing, to be started by next CIN meeting.	Olivia will be having a good experience at school and will be feeling calmer and more relaxed.
Mr and Mrs Green Jenni	Olivia is locked in her bedroom at night, which Mr and Mrs Green do because they have no alternative to keep her safe. Other options need to be explored, and occupational therapist consulted and a safety plan completed to ensure that Olivia is as safe as possible. Jenni will contact occupational health and the fire service to explore alternative methods; fire officer to undertake safety checks.	CIN meeting.	Olivia will be as safe as possible and everyone involved acknowledge, agree and sign a risk to safety assessment agreement. Risks of Olivia being locked in her bedroom at night are managed and reviewed.
Elaine Brown Mrs Green Sarah Sheen	Mrs Green and Sarah would like Olivia to be managing her continence and recommend a toileting programme to be in place. Elaine is supporting this and is going to meet with the setting and parents to start and review toileting programme.	CIN meeting.	Olivia will have a toileting programme in place that will be being followed by each setting.

» *Involvement of night nurse for specialist support with William's sleeping, behaviour management and routines.*

» *Continuing healthcare assessment undertaken and now providing one night per week support from carers (provided by Friendly Carers for consistency).*

» *Occupational therapy undertook an assessment for a safe area, including additional padding on bedroom walls and making safe windowsill and windows. Disabled Facilities Grant was agreed (see Chapter 9).*

We suggest you draw up a blank plan, perhaps using the same headings as the plan we have shown you, to keep it easy for you (or you could use a template you are more familiar with if you like) and then write your plan. Good luck.

Chapter 3: Managing the emotional impact of disability

Testing your emotional intelligence and resilience

Scenario: A brief life

Jessie is 18 months old and has a rare, life-limiting complex health condition. You have been involved since Jessie was eight months old and have been supporting her parents as they have both been in denial about her real prognosis. You have supported them in working with the hospice to formulate an Advanced Care Plan, which is a plan for end of life care.

You have walked in to work on a Monday morning to be given the sad news of Jessie's death, following a sudden severe episode where doctors were unable to resuscitate her. There are procedures to follow around visiting and supporting the family and despite her dying in hospital, the safeguarding policy requires a child death review; legislation that came out of previous serious case reviews rules that all children involved with Children's Services who die will have a child death review. As a professional you will be expected to be a strong support for the family through their grieving process and you may be asked to attend the funeral. You will be enabling the family to access financial support to help them with funeral costs and perhaps discussing plans and arrangements for the funeral with them.

How do you feel? Can you envisage some of the conversations you will be having with parents? Do you have the emotional intelligence to know when there does not need to be a conversation or words, and that just to be with someone on their difficult journey can say more than many words? How might you react, respond or feel in managing this situation for the first time?

This is something that no book or advice can prepare you for. It is your emotional intelligence that will carry you through the experience and enable you to follow your instincts about how you manage and continue to display strength for the family.

Chapter 4: The child's voice: exploring their world using good communication

Scenario: Liam, Liam, Liam…

Liam is nine years old and is diagnosed with autism. He has a good level of speech although this presents in the form of echolalia, where he will copy almost word by word what he hears and what you say to him. For example, if on a visit you ask him to say goodbye by saying 'Goodbye, Liam' he would repeat 'Goodbye Liam' to you. He is also able to recall sentences and comments that he may have heard at school, and will often even give the same tone that the teacher has said it in. For example, he may say 'Liam, please don't do that' or 'It's snack time Liam, Liam, wash hands now'.

Liam's mum Annie is getting frustrated with Liam due to his echolalia, and she talks to you on a visit about how hard it is to give him instructions to get ready in the morning in time for his taxi to arrive. Annie gives an example that she had tried to ask him to get washed and dressed and that he just kept repeating what she said but did not understand that it was an instruction. He remained sat on the bed repeating everything she said and when she got a bit cross with him he continued to repeat all of her words, even when she was then trying to ask him why he won't do as she asks. Annie says she understands about Liam having echolalia, but that she cannot understand why he does not do the things, when he is able to repeat very clearly. Liam also loves nursery rhymes and some simple songs and will repeat them over and over when he is feeling happy.

How can you support Annie with finding ways to get Liam to follow her instructions to get ready in the morning?

What strengths can you identify for Liam? How can you build on his strengths to help him follow some basic tasks?

Liam's dentist appointment

Staying with Liam's story, Annie has called to let you know that Liam needs to attend the dentist, and she is really worried about how she can explain this to him. She is worried that he will not be able to sit in the chair and let the dentist have a look at his tooth; she thinks Liam may have an abscess.

How can you support with this?

What tools are there that can help Liam to know where he will be going and what will happen to him there?

What visual tools and resources can you think of or find?

Tip: there may be colourful children's story books about going to the dentist, and when the character's name is read it could be changed to 'Liam is going to the dentist'. This could be read and Liam encouraged to repeat it. There could be dressing-up games to play to act out what a dentist would do when Liam lies back in a chair. Visits could be made to the dentist prior to the actual appointment where Liam can see the setting and meet the people there.

Chapter 5: Autism and its impact on communication

Scenario: Brad does not like clothes

Brad is eight years old with severe autism and has difficulty with social behaviour; he will often strip all his clothes off at school due to sensory needs and has no inhibitions about presenting naked in front of others as his main need and focus is the discomfort of the clothing next to his skin. He does not understand that this is not appropriate behaviour and it would be difficult to try and explain why to him. He has no verbal communication and will just make some sounds now and then.

What does his behaviour tell you? Is he expressing his views and needs and what might these be? How do you protect him from the vulnerability of exposing himself without any self-awareness around his own safety and dignity?

How can school help? What about the other vulnerable children in his group who are witness to this behaviour?

What research might you need to look at? Who else might you talk with to explore strategies?

Scenario: An older child's worrying behaviour

Darren is 17 years old and lives in supported living accommodation with four other young adults. Darren has Asperger's, epilepsy that is managed by medication, and mild learning disabilities.

Darren smokes and he is always asking the other residents for cigarettes. He also drinks alcohol, having approximately three cans of lager most evenings. He saves his money for the lager and also asks other residents for money to buy his lager and cigarettes. He sometimes goes off-site to the local bar and some of the regular customers feel sorry for Darren and buy him a drink, despite his only being 17 years old and under age.

When Darren has been drinking a lot he sometimes becomes aggressive towards the staff and other residents at the unit. He is often hung over the next morning and has been late for his supported apprenticeship: he has been given a verbal warning. If he loses this placement, he will not be able to stay at the supported living accommodation as a condition of living there is that Darren remains in his apprenticeship. Staff are worried about Darren's health due to his smoking and excessive drinking.

If you were Darren's social worker what would you do next? What conclusions have you drawn about Darren's situation? What do you think about Darren's mental capacity and his rights to drinking and smoking and the risk that he might lose his placement? How did you reach that decision? What about his behaviour towards staff and other residents? Who else was involved in your decision making?

Write a plan for a meeting that you have arranged for tomorrow. Consider how you will engage with Darren so that he understands your concerns.

Chapter 6: Completing your assessment

Scenario: Keeping siblings in focus

Ruth is 17 years old, diagnosed with Asperger's, and has acute anxiety related behaviours. When in a state of high anxiety, Ruth will display screaming, shouting, swearing and throwing things that are in her reach; cups and objects get thrown at her mother Patty, her siblings and anyone else who tries to intervene. Ruth does not discriminate about who gets hurt by the objects thrown or from her hitting out as her anxiety becomes her only focus. Even if her voice is becoming hoarse through the screaming and shouting, Ruth does not have an awareness of the harm she is doing to her throat and will continue until she is able to calm down again.

Ruth's anxieties stem from her transitions of sometimes leaving the house to go to respite or college. Even though she has been attending both settings regularly it is the actual leaving of the house that is the trigger. Ruth attends respite once per week.

Ruth has three siblings: Zoe age 12, Aiden age nine and Ella age 6. All three siblings have had most of their objects broken and only recently Zoe had her laptop thrown across the room when she brought it downstairs for her mum to help her with some homework.

Zoe, Aiden and Ella have taken to retreating to their bedrooms to stay out of the way of Ruth's outbursts, but more and more during increasingly frequent visits by the social worker, the siblings are found to be out of the way most of the time and do not come down to say hello any more. Patty is tearful on most visits and has been seen shouting back at Ruth, trying to get her to leave the house and get into the taxi, and this is proving more and more difficult each time.

What is life like for Zoe, Aiden and Ella?

Try to think about each sibling as an individual, taking into account their age and their own emotional well-being.

What effects might Ruth's disability related behaviours have on Zoe's education and home life? Ask the same question for Aiden and Ella.

How is Patty managing to support Ruth and her other children? What are the risks you have identified? What support can you explore for Zoe, Aiden and Ella?

Is the support and respite at the right level? Is it allowing any time for the siblings to be in a home free from conflict, are they able to have some time with each other, with their mum or on their own?

How can extended family members help – have they had a Family Group Conference?

Chapter 7: Exploring behaviour management techniques and strategies

Scenario: Leaving on a jet plane

For this activity we will return to the case scenario of Joe from Chapter 7. To remind you in brief:

Joe is ten years old with autism and had been identified by the educational psychologist as functioning at around four years old, which meant that some of the family's problems stemmed from his parents expecting him to behave like a ten-year-old. Joe's parents are worried as they are planning a special family holiday abroad in a month's time. They do not know whether to take Joe as he has never been on a plane before and this might cause him to display his behaviours, which they would find difficult to manage on a plane. They don't really want him to miss out on the holiday as they don't want to exclude him from such a special family event and not be in the holiday memories and photos.

How can you help Joe's parents to prepare him and to enable him to go on and enjoy the holiday?

Remember Joe cannot follow long instructions, so he needs things explained very simply and basically.

You might want to remind yourself about some of the techniques and tools that can be adapted and designed to help Joe know what will be happening and also what an airport and the inside of a plane might look like. Think about what visual tools you can support his parents to access.

Think about how you could take a step-by-step approach with Joe's parents to help introduce the concept of the journey, the airport, the new country, the hotel etc.

Joe continued – ADD

Due to some continued difficulties in trying to get Joe to focus for any length of time and with CAMHS becoming involved, it has been recognised that Joe also has attention deficit disorder (ADD), which is a key factor in why his development and cognitive functioning is delayed. Joe's ADD means that he has a very short attention span of only a minute to a few minutes at a time. This shows with him wanting to flit between different activities very quickly; he is unable to sit and play for any length of time, which would give his parents some breathing space. He will jump up and down excitedly as he has given his parents a DVD film to put on, only to run off to do something else even before the titles have finished and the film started. The film needs to stay on though, as he will come back to the television and stand and watch bits of it in between flitting to other things. This has become exhausting for his parents, who are now trying to adapt and understand the new diagnosis –they are looking into it and now realising and recognising how this has affected his learning and development.

How can you support his parents in finding strategies to help occupy Joe's short-term concentration span and to help him expand his concentration?

What games can you look up that help children to do this?

Chapter 8: Giving consideration to values, ethics, race and anti-discriminatory practice

Scenario: When parents struggle too

Mr and Mrs Singh are the parents of Kulvinder, who has autism and learning difficulties. They also have an older daughter who attends mainstream education and is an open case to the Children with Disabilities Team for support from Targeted Youth Support. Mrs Singh has mental health problems and learning difficulties; Mr Singh also has a mild degree of learning difficulties and is Mrs Singh's carer. The family lived in Low Town at the time.

Mr and Mrs Singh were having problems with their neighbours which continued over a period of six months. The situation deteriorated to the point where Mr Singh became depressed, and both he and his wife felt uncomfortable leaving their home. This was having an impact on Kulvinder accessing the community, and he told me that he felt sad as the neighbours stared at him and pointed.

The housing association agreed to send out a housing officer to look at a possible move to High Town for the family. This did not go well, however, and the housing officer was not very sympathetic about the family's circumstances; Mrs Singh admitted that she was rude to the housing officer and Mr Singh lost his temper, which did not help the situation.

The housing officer informs that the home conditions were poor, and they could not understand why there were locks on the doors of the front room, kitchen and a child's room.

While in the middle of all the trouble with the neighbours, how do you think the family are feeling about their place and acceptance in their community?

What values or discrimination do you draw from this situation? How can you help Mr and Mrs Singh move forward again? What about exploring Kulvinder's views further in relation to how he feels about the neighbours not being very nice and staring?

What things would you consider and what actions would you take about the lock on the door? (see Chapter 2 for help).

Remember to consider the sibling's views, too.

Chapter 9: Accessing support and resources

Scenario: Risk assessing

Rosie is eight years old and has epilepsy, which is not yet under control and so she can have seizures throughout the day or night. Rosie's mother Mandy is a lone carer and needs to monitor Rosie through the night, meaning she is sleep deprived. Mandy is isolated in that her extended family live away as she moved when her partner got a new job; however due to the pressure of caring for Rosie, he left her about six months ago. While she has been trying to manage on her own, she is starting to feel the strain and is presenting as tired and stressed.

What are the risks identified for Mandy to continue to care this way on her own?

What support have you identified?

Is there is an identified need for a support worker, perhaps through direct payments, to give Mandy an opportunity to recharge and be able to have at least one night of restful sleep? You will also need to help Mandy draw up a risk assessment in order that any support worker knows what do to in the event of a seizure.

Chapter 10: Exploring a family perspective

The qualities of good and bad social workers

Having read this chapter and considered the family perspectives we would like you to think about your own practice: can you see in yourself any of the points discussed by the family members who were interviewed – good or bad? Be honest!

For a moment think about a social worker you know who you would NOT want to be working with your family, for example, if a referral was received about your own mother, father, sister, brother, or even your own child. What are the attributes and qualities of that worker that you do not think are very good? What makes you not want them knocking at your door and why? What has made you reach that conclusion? What have you witnessed that worker do or say that you did not like or feel was not very professional and you would not want him/her to say to you?

Now make a list of those attributes that you do not want to model in your practice ...

Now, in stark contrast we hope, think about a social worker that you know, perhaps in your team, who you *would* want to be allocated your own family's case.

What makes that person a good social worker? What are their qualities and attributes that make you think you would want to model your practice upon? What do you think they would do to make you or your family feel comfortable with them as their allocated social worker? What good practice have you seen that person do that makes you rate them as a social worker?

Make a list of those qualities that you want to model your practice on and aspire to be like ...

Having made your two lists and taken into consideration what parents believe make a good social worker, think about how you can put those good qualities into your own practice and if you have recognised any of the negative attributes in yourself. How are you going to change your practice to be more like the good social workers? How can you make this happen? Do you need to ask if you can shadow your selected good social worker? Complete the box below and use it as your plan of action.

What are the areas of my practice that I do not really like or want to change?	How do I ensure I make those changes?	What are the positive attributes I want to aspire to achieve?	How do I make it happen?

Glossary

ADD	Attention deficit disorder
ADHD	Attention deficit hyperactivity disorder
Anxiety disorder	a condition in which the sufferer experiences feelings of fear, being overwhelmed and worrying all the time
Aphasia	is a combination of speech and language disorder
ASD	Autistic spectrum disorder
Bereavement	a term used to describe the sense of loss felt when a loved one passes away
Bipolar disorder	is also known as bipolar affective disorder or manic depression, and is a mental disorder characterised by alternating periods of elevated mood and depression
BME	Black and Ethnic Minority
CAF	Common Assessment Framework, a standardised approach to conducting an assessment of a child's additional needs
CAMHS	Child and Adolescent Mental Health Services
CAPD	Central auditory processing disorder is a common hearing problem in children that can affect speech and learning
CCPNR	Children's Community Psychiatric Nurse
CDC	The Council for Disabled Children
Cerebral palsy	a condition that affects a child's ability to control their muscles. There are three types: spastic; athetoid (dyskinetic); and ataxic
CIN	Child in need, defined as a child with a disability or deemed to require the services of a local authority
CP	Child Protection (in medical settings the abbreviation could mean cerebral palsy)
CP	Community paediatrician
CTH	Ceiling track hoist, used to help move those with physical disabilities
CWD	Children with disabilities
DCD	Developmental co-ordination disorder, for example dyspraxia

DCSF	Department for Children, Schools and Families, which existed 2007-2010.
Depression	a psychiatric disorder characterised by low mood, anxiety, feelings of worthlessness, deep sadness, always seeing the worst-case scenario and thoughts of suicide or self-harming behaviour
Developmental receptive language disorder	a difficulty in understanding general speech and language.
DfE	Department for Education
DFG	Disabled Facilities Grant
DH	Department of Health
Disintegrative disorder	a condition where regression and loss of skills follow a period of normal development.
Down's syndrome	is a randomly occurring genetic condition caused by the presence of an extra chromosome. The severity varies, but Down's syndrome is associated with learning disabilities and delayed physical development.
DP	Direct Payment, made by local Health and Social Care Trusts to those in need who prefer to arrange and pay for their own care or support services as opposed to receiving them directly from the trust.
Dysgraphia	a neurological disorder characterised by difficulty in creating legible handwriting.
Dyslexia	a learning difficulty associated with problems in spelling and writing words, reading quickly, 'sounding out' words in the head, pronouncing words when reading aloud and understanding what one reads.
Dysphagia	a swallowing disorder in which a person may have problems swallowing certain foods or liquids, or be unable to swallow at all.
Dysphasia	a language disorder whereby a person has full or partial loss of speech and communication skills, sometimes including comprehending others.
Dyspraxia	a common form of developmental co-ordination disorder (DCD) affecting fine and/or gross motor co-ordination in children and adults. It may also affect speech.

EBD	Emotional and behaviour difficulty
Echolalia	a condition associated with autism involving the repetition of words or phrases immediately after a word or sentence is said.
EEG	Electroencephalogram, a procedure for measuring the brain's electrical activity to record the natural activity of the brain.
EFA	Education Funding Agency
EHC Plan	Education, Health and Care Plan, for children and adults up to the age of 25 with SEND.
EHE	Elective home education, when parents decide to educate their child(ren) at home instead of sending them to school.
Epilepsy	a neurological condition characterised by abnormal electrical activity in the brain causing seizures.
EP	Educational psychologist
EPO	Emergency protection order
EWO	Education Welfare Officer
EYFS	Early Years Foundation Stage, covers standards for the care and education of children from birth to five years old.
FAS	Foetal alcohol syndrome is the direct result of alcohol exposure due to an expectant mother's drinking, particularly during the first trimester. Children affected can suffer neurological problems, including learning difficulties, and physical issues.
Frontal lobes	the front parts of the cerebral hemispheres of the brain, responsible for many higher cognitive functions (complex reasoning, thinking and planning ahead, for example).
GDD	Global developmental delay is the term used to describe when a child has not met their 'expected' developmental milestones. The delay may be more significant for some children than others, with some having severe communication difficulties and other additional learning disabilities.
GP	General practitioner
HI	Hearing impaired
Hydrocephalus	a build-up of cerebrospinal fluid (CSF) on the brain, which may be treated by a shunt to drain the fluid. If left untreated can in some circumstances be fatal.
Hyperkinetic disorder	extreme hyperactivity and repetitive behaviour

IEP	Individual Education Plan, designed to help children with special educational needs get the most out of their education.
ICPCC	Initial Child Protection Case Conference
Joint hypermobility	means that a person has a large range of movement in their joints, but this can be painful and they can be prone to dislocation. The condition can also be associated with fatigue, dizziness and digestive problems.
Ketogenic diet	often used to treat children with epilepsy, and consists of high fat, adequate protein and low carbohydrates.
Kidney disease	including chronic kidney disease (CKD), a long-term condition that may require dialysis or a kidney transplant.
KS	Key Stage, a classification system for expected levels of knowledge in children.
LA	Local authority
LAC	Looked-After Children are under the care of a local authority for more than 24 hours.
LADO	Local Authority Designated Officer, an employee who manages any concerns about staff or volunteers with regard to child safety.
LAS	Level access shower, a walk-in shower without any sort of step or ledge, to aid those with mobility issues.
LD	Learning disability
LEA	Local Education Authority
Limbic system	a group of interlinked brain structures responsible for aspects of emotional, sexual and eating behaviour.
LLDD	Learners with learning difficulties or disabilities
M&H	Moving and handling of people with physical impairments
MAM	Multi-agency meeting, a meeting of representatives from different agencies to discuss eg a Common Assessment.
MD	Muscular dystrophy. A group of inherited progressive genetic conditions, more commonly affecting boys, which cause the muscles to weaken over time, leading to increasing disability and often early death. There are various types, including Duchenne's, myotonic and facioscapulohumeral.
MLD	Moderate learning difficulty

MS	Multiple sclerosis is a progressive or relapsing autoimmune condition, usually developing in the 20s or 30s, in which the body attacks the nervous system, causing neurological and physical symptoms.
NAS	National Autistic Society
NINDS	the National Institute of Neurological Disorders and Stroke
NOFAS-UK	National Organisation for Foetal Alcohol Syndrome
NSPCC	National Society for the Prevention of Cruelty to Children
NVLD	Non-verbal learning disorder (or non-verbal learning disability), characterised by verbal strengths but visual-spatial, motor and social difficulties.
NWB	Non-weight bearing, when no weight can be placed on a lower extremity.
OCD	Obsessive Compulsive Disorder is a mental health condition which manifests by a child or adult having obsessive thoughts and compulsive, often repetitive, activity.
Ofsted	Office for Standards in Education
OT	Occupational therapist
Optician	dispenses lenses and frames, ensuring they fit correctly
Optometrist	a specialist in the diagnosis and treatment of visual refractive errors
Orthoptist	specialists in the diagnosis and treatment of ocular motility disorders, ocular misalignments and amblyopia ('lazy eye'). They specialise in correcting vision by non-surgical means.
Ophthalmologist	a physician who specialises in eye diseases and eye defects and who uses surgery and medicine to manage eye conditions.
Palliative care	medical care provided by specially trained health professionals for people with serious illnesses, which is often end of life care.
PD	Physical disability
PMLD	Profound and multiple learning difficulties
PR	Parental responsibility
Prosthesis	artificial limb
PRU	Pupil Referral Unit, sometimes known as a Pupil Re-integration Unit, a local authority establishment that provides education for children who are unable to attend a mainstream school.

PT	Physiotherapy
SALT	Speech and language therapy, used in a variety of settings with children and young people who have identified Speech, Language and Communication Needs (SLCN) and/or motor difficulties with eating, drinking or swallowing.
SB	Spina bifida, a common birth defect characterised by a gap in the spine, which can cause paralysis and incontinence. It can be associated with hydrocephalus, which may lead to learning difficulties.
SCA	Social care assessment
Scoliosis	an abnormal twisting or curve of the spine, often creating a C or an S shape. It usually develops between the ages of 10-15.
SENCO	Special Educational Needs Coordinator
SEND	Special Educational Needs and Disability
SLD	Severe Learning Difficulty
SOS	Signs of Safety, a model for child protection based on collaboration with families and children to reduce risk.
SpLD	Specific learning difficulties
Specialist Nurse Trainers	nurses with qualifications in children's nursing that have a range of experience in caring for children with disabilities both in the community and in hospital settings.
Stroke	a common condition caused when the blood flow to the brain is disrupted. Some are very mild, but others can cause speech and mobility problems, and some are fatal.
TA	Teaching assistant
TAC	Team Around the Child, a multi-agency meeting to discuss any concerns about a child or young person with additional needs.
TFL	Through floor lift
Tourette's syndrome	The diagnosis of Tourette's syndrome occurs when both motor and phonic tics are experienced over at least 12 months. It is a neurological condition that affects the brain and nervous system, characterised by 'tics' – involuntary noises (coughing, grunting or shouting words, often obscene) or involuntary movements. It can be associated with OCD and ADHD.
UPN	Unique Pupil Number, an identification number that stays with a child throughout their time at school.

VI	Visually impaired
Visual Processing Disorder	a sensory disability related to the processing of images
VNS	Vagal (or vagus) nerve stimulation is a medical treatment that involves delivering electrical impulses to the vagus nerve, used to treat epilepsy and depression when other treatments have failed.
X	Fragile X syndrome is the most common known cause of inherited learning disabilities, more prevalent in boys. Children show autistic-like features, including: avoiding eye contact, anxiety in social situations, insistence on familiar routines and hand flapping or hand biting.
XXY	AKA Klinefelter syndrome is a genetic condition that only affects boys, who are born with an extra X chromosome. Girls with an extra X chromosome have what is called Triple X syndrome. In Klinefelter's there are low testosterone levels, and it can be associated with mild learning difficulties and problems socialising. Triple X syndrome can cause delayed development of motor skills and learning/speech difficulties.
YOS	Youth Offending Service (formerly YOT – Youth Offending Team)

References

Abbott, D, Morris, J and Ward, L (2001) *The best place to be? Policy, practice and the experiences of residential school placements for disabled children.* Joseph Rowntree Foundation.

Adams, J and Sheard, A (2013) *Positive Social Work: The Essential Toolkit for NQSWs.* St Albans: Critical Publishing Ltd.

Barn, R (2006) 'Improving services to meet the needs of minority ethnic children and families' Briefing Paper 13 Research in Practice. Making Research Count. London. Department of Health www.rip.org.uk/resources/publications/frontline-resources/improving-services-to-meet-the-needs-of-minority-ethnic-children-and-families-.

Barnes, C and Mercer, G (2004) *Implementing the social model of disability: Theory and Research.* Leeds: The Disability Press.

Baron-Cohen, S, Tager-Flusberg, H, Cohen, D J (eds) (1994) *Understanding other minds: Perspectives from Autism.* New York: Oxford University Press, pp xiii 515. Available online http://psycnet.apa.org/psycinfo/1993-98373-000 (accessed 30 September 2015).

Bartlett, P, Hussain, T, Hyde-Bales, K, Killwick, P, Pointu, A, Seale, K and Shaw, S (2015) *Independent review into issues that may have contributed to the preventable death of Connor Sparrowhawk. A report for: NHS England, South Region Oxfordshire Safeguarding Adults Board.* London: Verita.

Bennett, H (August 2012) *A Guide to End of Life Care: Care of children and young people before death, at the time of death and after death.* Bristol: Together for Short Lives. Available online www.togetherforshortlives.org.uk (accessed 25 April 2015).

Block, R W and Krebs, N F, the Committee on Child Abuse and Neglect and the Committee on Nutrition (2005) Failure to Thrive as a Manifestation of Child Neglect, *Pediatrics* Vol. 116 No. 5, pp. 1234–1237 (doi: 10.1542/peds.2005–2032). Available online http://pediatrics.aappublications.org/content/116/5/1234.full (accessed 26 April 2015).

Boddy, J, Potts, P and Stratham, J (2006) *Models of good practice in joined-up assessment: Working for children with significant and complex needs.* Research. London: London School of Economics. Available online www.ccinform.co.uk/research/models-of-good-practice-in-joined-up-assessment-working-for-children-with-significant-and-complex-needs/ (accessed 11 February 2015).

Brandon, M, Bailey, S, Belderson, P, Gardner, R, Sidebottom, P, Dodsworth, J, Warren, C and Black, J (2009) *Understanding Serious Case Reviews and their impact: A Biennial Analysis of Serious Case Reveiws 2005–7.* London: Department for Children Schools and Families.

Bronfenbrenner, U (1977) Toward an experimental ecology of human development. *American Psychologist*, 32, 513–531.

Clements, L and Read, J (2003) *Disabled People and European Human Rights.* Bristol: The Policy Press.

Collins, M, Langer, S, Welch, V, Wells, E, Hatton, C, Robertson, J and Emerson, E (2009) *An initial report on preliminary themes emerging form qualitative research into the impact of short break provision on families with disabled children.* Lancaster: Centre for Disability Research (CeDR)/Lancaster University.

Department for Children, Schools and Families (2008) *Special Educational Needs in England.* London: DCSF.

Department for Children, Schools and Families (2008a) *Aiming High for Disabled Children: Transforming services for disabled children and their families.* Nottingham: DCSF Publications.

Department for Children, Schools and Families (2008b) *Children in whom illness is fabricated or induced. Supplementary Guidance to Working Together to Safeguard Children.* London DCSF. Available online www.gov.uk/government/uploads/system/uploads/attachment_data/file/277314/Safeguarding_Children_in_whom_illness_is_fabricated_or_induced.pdf (accessed 27 December 2015).

Department for Children, Schools and Families and Department of Health (2008) *Aiming High for Disabled Children: Short breaks implementation guidance.* London: DH.

Department for Children, Schools and Families (2009) *Safeguarding Disabled Children: Practice guidance.* Nottingham: DCSF.

Department for Children, Schools and Families (DCSF) (2010) *Working Together to Safeguard Children: A Guide to Inter-Agency Working to safeguard and promote the welfare of children.* London: DCSF.

Department for Children, Schools and Families (DCSF) (2010a) *Short Breaks Statutory Guidance on how to safeguard and promote the welfare of disabled children using short breaks.* London: DCSF.

Department for Children Schools and Families (DCSF) (2010b) *The Children Act 1989 Guidance and Regulations Volume 2: Care Planning, Placement and Case Review.* Nottingham: DCSF Publications. Available online www.gov.uk/government/uploads/system/uploads/attachment_data/file/336072/The_Children_Act_1989_Care_planning_placement_case_review.pdf (accessed 23 August 2015).

Department for Children Schools and Families (DCSF) (2010c) *IRO Handbook Statutory guidance for independent reviewing officers and local authorities on their functions in relation to case management and review.* DCSF Nottingham. Available online www.gov.uk/government/uploads/system/uploads/attachment_data/file/337568/iro_statutory_guidance_iros_and_las_march_2010_tagged.pdf (accessed 10 January 2016).

Department for Education (2011) An Action Plan for Adoption: Tackling Delay. DfE. Available online www.gov.uk/government/uploads/system/uploads/attachment_data/file/180250/action_plan_for_adoption.pdf. You can also download this booklet online at: http://publications.education.gov.uk/ (accessed 10 May 2015).

Department for Education (2011a) *Short breaks for carers of disabled children: Departmental advice for local authorities.* London: DfE. Available online www.gov.uk/government/uploads/system/uploads/attachment_data/file/245580/Short_Breaks_for_Carers_of_Disabled_Children.pdf. You can also download this online at: www.gov.uk/government/publications (accessed 1 August 2015).

Department for Education (2013) *Working Together to Safeguard Children: A guide to inter-agency working to safeguard and promote the welfare of children.* London: DFE. Available online www.education.gov.uk/aboutdfe/statutory (accessed 16 May 2015).

Department for Education (2013b) *School Funding Reform: Findings from the Review of Arrangements and Changes for 2014/15.* London: DfE.

Department for Education (2014) Supported internships: Advice for further education colleges, sixth forms in academies, maintained and non-maintained schools independent specialist providers, other providers of study programmes and local authorities. Available online www.gov.uk/government/uploads/system/uploads/attachment_data/file/389411/Supported_Internship_Guidance_Dec_14.pdf (accessed 11 December 2015).

Department for Education (2014a) The *Children Act 1989 Guidance and Regulations Volume 3: planning transition to adulthood for care leavers* (revision date January 2015) London: DfE. Available online www.gov.uk/government/uploads/system/uploads/attachment_data/file/397649/CA1989_Transitions_guidance.pdf (accessed 9 August 2015).

Department for Education and Department of Health (2015) *Special Educational Needs and Disability Code of Practice: 0 to 25 years. Statutory guidance for organisations which work with and support children and young people who have special educational needs or disabilities.* London: DfE. Available online www.gov.uk/government/uploads/system/uploads/attachment_data/file/398815/SEND_Code_of_Practice_January_2015.pdf (accessed 25 August 2015).

Department for Education (2015) *Working together to safeguard children: A guide to inter-agency working to safeguard and promote the welfare of children.* London: DfE. Available online www.workingtogetheronline.co.uk/; www.gov.uk/government/uploads/system/uploads/attachment_data/file/419595/Working_Together_to_Safeguard_Children.pdf (accessed 27 December 2015).

Department for Education and Skills (DfES) (2004) *Monitoring protocol for deaf babies and children Level 2 materials.* Nottingham: DfES.

Department for Education and Skills (DfES) (2004a) *Information for parents: visual impairment.* Nottingham: DfES.

The Department for Education and Skills (2006) Every Child Matters: Change for children agenda. Available online www.rip.org.uk/publications/researchbriefings.asp (accessed 30 November 2015).

Department of Constitutional Affairs (2007) Mental Capacity Act 2005 Code of Practice. Birmingham: Office of the Public Guardian. Available online www.gov.uk/government/uploads/system/uploads/attachment_data/file/224660/Mental_Capacity_Act_code_of_practice.pdf (accessed 19 January 2016).

Department of Health (2000) *Assessing children in need and their families: practice guidance.* London: The Stationery Office.

Department of Health (2001) *Valuing People: A New Strategy for Learning Disability for the 21st Century, White Paper.* London: Stationery Office.

Department of Health (2002) *Planning with People Towards Person-Centred Approaches: Guidance for Partnership Boards.* London: DoH.

Department of Health (2003) Local Authority Circular LAC (2003) 14. London: DoH. Available online http://webarchive.nationalarchives.gov.uk/20130107105354/http://www.dh.gov.uk/prod_consum_dh/groups/dh_digitalassets/@dh/@en/documents/digitalasset/dh_4012833.pdf (accessed 15 November 2015).

Department of Health (2004) *National Service Framework for Children, Young People and Maternity Services.* London: DoH.

Department of Health (2006) *Working Together to Safeguard Children: A guide to inter- agency working to safeguard and promote the welfare of children.* London: TSO.

Department of Health (2007) *Good practice guidance on working with parents with a learning disability.* London: DoH and DfES http://webarchive.nationalarchives.gov.uk/20080910224541/dh.gov.uk/en/Publicationsandstatistics/Publications/PublicationsPolicyAndGuidance/DH_075119 (accessed 26 April 2015).

Department of Health (2008) *Better Communication: Improving Services for Children and Young People with Speech, Language and Communication Needs.* London: DoH.

Department of Health (2009) *Guidance on Direct Payment for Community Care, Services for Carers and Children's Services.* London: DoH.

Department of Health (2010) *Fulfilling and rewarding lives: The strategy for adults with autism in England.* London: DoH. Available online http://webarchive.nationalarchives.gov.uk/20130107105354/http://www.dh.gov.uk/prod_consum_dh/groups/dh_digitalassets/@dh/@en/@ps/documents/digitalasset/dh_113405.pdf (accessed 12 October 2015).

Department of Health (2010a) *National Framework for Children and Young People's Continuing Care.* London: DoH. Available online www.cen.scot.nhs.uk/files/11b-national-framework-for-continuing-care-england.pdf (accessed 15 December 2015).

Department of Health (2010b) *National Framework for Children and Young People's Continuing Care.* London: DoH. Available online www.gov.uk/government/uploads/system/uploads/attachment_data/file/499611/children_s_continuing_care_Fe_16.pdf (accessed 21 March 2016).

Department of Health (2011) *Health Visitor Implementation Plan 2011–2015: A Call to Action.* London: DoH.

Department of Health (2014) *Care Act 2014 Chapter 23 Part 1 – Care and Support.* London: TSO.

Department of Health (2014b) *Care and Support Statutory Guidance Issued under the Care Act 2014 Department of Health.* London: DoH.

Department of Health (2014c) *Children and Families Act Chapter 6.* London: TSO. Available online www.legislation.gov.uk/ukpga/2014/6/pdfs/ukpga_20140006_en.pdf (accessed 22 August 2015).

Dworzynski, K, Ronald, A, Bolton, P and Happé, F (2012) How different are girls and boys above and below the diagnostic threshold for autism spectrum disorders? *J Am Acad Child Adolesc Psychiatry* Aug;51(8):788–97.

Education Funding Agency (2014) *Schools revenue funding 2015 to 2016: Operational Guide.* London: Education Funding Agency (EFA). Available online www.gov.uk/government/uploads/system/uploads/attachment_data/file/414929/Schools_revenue_funding_2015_to_2016_operational_guide_March_2015.pdf (accessed 2 September 2015).

Emmerson, E (2001) *Challenging Behaviour: Analysis and Intervention in People with Severe Intellectual Disabilities.* Cambridge: Cambridge University Press.

Evans, M and Whittaker, A (2010) *Sensory Awareness and Social Work.* Exeter: Learning Matters.

4Children (2013) Best Practice for a Sure Start: The Way Forward for Children's Centres. www.4children.org.uk/Files/cffc42fe-49eb-43e2-b330-a1fd00b8077b/Best-Practice-for-a-Sure-Start.pdf (accessed 20 November 2015).

4Children (2014) Children & Family Hubs: 4Children's integrated model for effective children and family support. www.4children.org.uk/Files/e49c7544-413b-4273-a979-a3e900b913a3/ChildrenFamilyHubs Model.pdf (accessed 20 November 2015).

Family Rights Group Family group conferences www.frg.org.uk/involving-families/family-group-conferences (accessed 15 December 2015).

Fraser et al (2011) *Life-Limiting Conditions in Children in the UK*, Division of Epidemiology. Leeds: University of Leeds.

General Medical Council (2010) *Treatment and care towards the end of life: good practice in decision making.* Manchester: General Medical Council. Available online www.gmc-uk.org (accessed 26 April 2015).

Goleman, D (1996) *Emotional Intelligence: Why it can matter more than IQ.* London: Bloomsbury.

Goleman, D (1998) *Working with emotional intelligence.* New York: Bantam Books.

Grandin, T (1995) *Thinking in pictures: And other reports from my life with autism.* New York: Doubleday.

Hasson, G. (2012) *Brilliant Emotional Intelligence: Harness the power of emotions; succeed in all areas of your life*, Harlow: Pearson Education Limited.

Hatton, C, Collins, M, Welch, V, Robertson, J, Emerson, E, Langer, S and Wells, E (2011) *The impact of short breaks on families with a disabled child over time: The second report from the quantitative study. Executive Summary.* London: DfE. Available online www.gov.uk/government/uploads/system/uploads/attachment_data/file/197641/DFE-RBX-10–12.pdf; www.gov.uk/government/uploads/system/uploads/attachment_data/ file/417669/Archived-Working_together_to_safeguard_children.pdf (accessed 1 August 2015).

Healy, K (2005) *Social Work Theories in Context.* Basingstoke: Palgrave Macmillan.

H M Government (HM Govt) (2011) *Prevent Strategy.* Norwich: TSO. Available online www.gov.uk/government/uploads/system/uploads/attachment_data/file/97976/prevent-strategy-review.pdf (accessed 24 January 2016).

Horwath, J (2001) *The Child's World: Assessing Children in Need.* London: Jessica Kingsley Publishers Ltd.

Howe, D (2008) *The Emotionally Intelligent Social Worker.* Hampshire: Palgrave Macmillan.

Jacobs, M (1989) *Psychodynamic Counselling in Action.* London: Sage Publications.

Jones, D P H (2003) *Communicating with vulnerable children: a guide for practitioners.* London: Gaskell.

Kao, B, Plante, W, and Lobato, D (2009) The use of the Impact on Sibling scale with families of children with chronic illness and development disability. *Child: Care, Health and Development*, 35(4), pp 505–509.

Available online www.scie-socialcareonline.org.uk/the-use-of-the-impact-on-sibling-scale-with-families-of-children-with-chronic-illness-and-developmental-disability/r/a1CG0000000GSnPMAW (accessed 22 April 2015).

Koprowska, J (2006) *Communication and Interpersonal Skills in Social Work*. Exeter: Learning Matters.

Kubler-Ross, E (1973) *On Death and Dying*. London: Routledge.

Kubler-Ross, E and Kessler, D (2014) *On Grief and Grieving: Finding the Meaning of Grief Through the Five Stages of Loss*, New York: Scribner.

Langer, S, Collins, M, Welch, V, Wells, E, Hatton, C, Robertson, J and Emerson, E (2010) *A Report on Themes Emerging from Qualitative Research into the Impact of Short Break Provision on Families with Disabled Children. Research Report DCSF – RR221*. Department for Children Schools and Families & Centre for Disability Research, Lancaster University, London, UK. Available online www.education.gov.uk/publications/standard/publicationdetail/page1/DCSF-RR221 (accessed 1 August 2015).

Maclean, S and Harrison, R (2008) *Social Work Theory. A Straightforward Guide for Practice Assessors and Placement Supervisors*. Rugeley: Kirwin Maclean Associates Limited.

Mencap (2007) *Death by indifference: Following up the Treat me right! Report*. London: Mencap. Available online www.pmldnetwork.org/resources/death_indifference_report_easyread.pdf (accessed 2 January 2016).

Merchant, R (1991) Myths and facts about sexual abuse and children with disabilities, *Child Abuse Reviews*, 5.2, pp 22–24. (Cited in Department for Children, Schools and Families (2009) Safeguarding Disabled Children: Practice guidance. Nottingham: DCSF, p 49.)

Mesibov, G B, Shea, V and Schopler, E (2004) *The TEACCH approach to autism spectrum disorders (Issues in Child Psychology)*. New York: Springer.

Minnis, M. and Walker, F. (2012) *The Experiences of Fostering and Adoption Processes – the Views of Children and Young People: Literature Review and Gap Analysis*. Slough: NFER.

Mitchell, W, Franklin, A, Greco, V and Bell, M (2009) Working with children with learning disabilities and/or who communicate non-verbally: research experiences and their implications for social work education, increased participation and social inclusion. *Social Work Education*, 28, 3 pp 309–324.

Munro, E (2011) *The Munro Review of Child Protection: Final Report – A child-centred system*. London: TSO. Available online www.gov.uk/government/uploads/system/uploads/attachment_data/file/175391/Munro-Review.pdf (accessed 11 August 2015).

Murray, M and Osborne C and The Children's Society (2009) *Safeguarding Disabled Children: Practice Guidance*. Nottingham: The Children's Society: DCSF Publications. Available online www.gov.uk/government/publications?keywords=safeguarding+disabled+children&publication_filter_option=all&topics%5B%5D=all&departments%5B%5D=department-foreducation&official_document_status=all&world_locations%5B%5D=all&from_date=&to_date= and www.teachernet.gov.uk/publications (accessed 4 April 2015).

National Institute for Health and Care Excellence (NICE) (2011) Autism diagnosis in children and young people. Recognition, referral and diagnosis of children and young people on the autism spectrum. NICE clinical guideline 128. www.guidance.nice.org.uk/cg128 (accessed 3 October 2015).

NHS South Central (2010) Child and Young Persons Advanced Care Plan Policy. Available online www.southcentral.nhs.uk (accessed 25 April 2015).

Osbourne, C (2011) Protecting disabled children from abuse and neglect, *Personnel Today*. Available online www.communitycare.co.uk/2011/11/03/protecting-disabled-children-from-abuse-and-neglect/ (accessed 2 January 2016).

Paul, A and Cawson, P (2002) Safeguarding Disabled Children in Residential Settings: What We Know and What We Don't Know, *Child Abuse Review*, Vol 11, pp 262–281.

Prizant, B, Wetherby, A, Rubin, E, Laurent, A and Rydell, P (2006) *The SCERTS Model: A Comprehensive*

Educational Approach for Children with Autism Spectrum Disorders. Baltimore, MD: Paul H Brookes Publishing.

Radcliffe, J J L and Turk, V (2008) Distress in children with learning disabilities at a respite unit: perspectives on their experiences, *British Journal of Learning Disabilities* Vol 36, Issue 2 91–101.

RNIB (2011) *Visual Impairment Speech and Language Therapy Best of Both: working together to support children with visual impairments and additional complex needs.* Leaflet PR12322P: RNIB.

Robertson, J, Hatton, C, Emerson, E, Wells, E, Collins, M, Langer, S and Welch, V (2009) *The impact of short breaks provision on disabled children and families: an international literature review.* Lancaster: Centre for Disability Research (CeDR), Lancaster University.

Robinson, C, Jackson, P and Townsley, R (2001) Short breaks for families caring for a disabled child with complex health needs, *Child and Family Social Work* Vol 6, 67–75.

Salmon, K (2015) Information adapted from workshop title: Understanding behaviour & low arousal approach. Held on 18 November 2015 at Sleaford.

Sheppard, M (1995) Social Work, Social Science and Practice Wisdom, *British Journal of Social Work* 25(3): 265–293.

Sheppard, M (2006) *Social Work and Social Exclusion.* Aldershot: Ashgate Publishing Limited.

Shore, S M (2004) Perception, *SI Focus Magazine* summer edn, pp 17–19. Available online www.cmcgc.com/media/handouts/101103/220_Stephen_Shore.pdf (accessed 10 October 2015).

Smith-Myles, B, Cook, K, Miller, N, Rinner, L and Robbins, L (2000) *Asperger Syndrome and Sensory Issues: Practical solutions for making sense of the world.* Shawnee Mission: KS: Autism Asperger Publishing Company.

Social Care, Local Government and Care Partnership Directorate, Department of Health (2014) *THINK AUTISM Fulfilling and Rewarding Lives, the strategy for adults with autism in England: an update.* London: H M Government. Available online www.gov.uk/government/uploads/system/uploads/attachment_data/file/299866/Autism_Strategy.pdf (accessed 12 October 2015).

Social Care, Local Government and Care Partnerships, Mental Health and Disability and Dementia (2015) *Statutory guidance for Local Authorities and NHS organisations to support implementation of the Adult Autism Strategy.* London: DoH.

Spivack, R, Craston, M, Graham, T and Carr, C (2014) Special Educational Needs and Disability Pathfinder Programme Evaluation Thematic Report: The Education, Health and Care (EHC) Planning Pathway for families that are new to the SEN system. Research Report. London: Department for Education. Available online www.gov.uk/government/publications (accessed 8 June 2015).

Stalker K, Green Lister, P, Lerpiniere J, McArthur, K (2010), *Child protection and the needs and rights of disabled children and young people: A scoping study*, Strathclyde: University of Strathclyde. Available online www.strathprints.strath.ac.uk/27036 (accessed 2 January 2016).

Standard Note (SN/SP/3011), Wilson W (2013) *Disabled Facilities Grants (England).* London: Social Policy Section, House of Commons.

Statutory Instruments (SI) (2009) *The Community Care Services for Carers and Children's Services (Direct Payments) (England) Regulations 2009, No 1887.* London: TSO.

Stroebe, M and Schut, H (1999) The Dual Process Model of Coping with Bereavement: Rationale and Description, *Death Studies*, 23:3, 197–224. Available online www.dx.doi.org/10.1080/074811899201046 (accessed 30 May 2015).

Stuart, M and Baines, C (2004) *Safeguards for vulnerable children.* Joseph Rowntree Foundation.

Sullivan P M and Knutson J F (2000) Maltreatment and disabilities: A population-based epidemiological study, *Child Abuse and Neglect*, 24, pp 1257–1273.

Swain, J, Finkelstein, V, French, S and Oliver, M (1993) *Disabling Barriers – Enabling Environments*, London: Sage Publications Ltd.

The Childhood Bereavement Network (CBN) for those working with bereaved children, young people and their families across the UK. www.childhoodbereavementnetwork.org.uk.

The Department for Communities and Local Government and Home Adaptations Consortium (2013) Delivering Housing Adaptations for Disabled People. A Detailed Guide to Related Legislation, Guidance and Good Practice. The Home Adaptations Consortium. http://careandrepair-england.org.uk/wp-content/uploads/2014/12/DFG-Good-Practice-Guide-30th-Sept-13.pdf (accessed 17 October 2015).

The National Deaf Children's Society (NCDS) 2002 *Deaf Friendly Schools: A Guide for Principals, Staff & Governors*. Belfast: NCDS.

The National Society for the Prevention of Cruelty to Children (NSPCC) (2003) *It Doesn't Happen to Disabled Children: Child Protection and Disabled Children. Report of the National Working Group on Child Protection and Disability*: London NSPCC.

The Office for Disability Issues, H M Government. Information available at www.dayjob.com/content/office-for-disability-issues-158.htm (accessed 9 November 2015).

Thomas, D and Woods, H (2006) *Working with People with Learning Disabilities Theory and Practice*, London: Jessica Kingsley Publishers.

Thomson, B (2013) *Non-Directive Coaching: Attitudes, Approaches and Applications*, St Albans: Critical Publishing Ltd.

Thompson, N (2006) *Anti-discriminatory Practice.* Basingstoke: Palgrave Macmillan.

Trevithick, P (2006) *Social Work Skills. A Practice Handbook*. Maidenhead: Open University Press.

Turnell, A and Edwards, S (1999) *Signs of Safety: A Solution and Safety Oriented Approach to Child Protection Casework*. New York: W.W. Norton.

Turnell, A and Essex, S (2006) *Working with 'Denied' Child Abuse: The Resolutions Approach*, Open University Press.

Turnell, A and Murphy, T (2014) *Signs of Safety: Child Protection Approach and Framework: 3rd Edition*. Australia: Resolutions Consultancy www.signsofsafety.net (accessed 9 October 2015).

Tutt, R, Powell, S D and Thornton, M (2006) Educational approaches in autism: what we know about what we do. *Educational Psychology in Practice* Vol 22, pp 69–81.

Unicef (2012) *A Better Life for Everyone. A Summary of the UN Convention on the Rights of the Child*. London: Unicef UK www.unicef.org.uk/Documents/Publication-pdfs/betterlifeleaflet2012_press.pdf (accessed 26 September 2015).

Utting, W. (1997) *People Like Us: The Report of the Review of Safeguards for Children Living Away from Home*. London: HMSO.

Weisler, S E and Milekic, S (1999) *Theory of Language*. Cambridge Massachusetts: MIT Press.

Welch, V, Hatton, C, Wells, E, Collins, M, Langer, S, Robertson, J and Emerson, E (2010) *The impact of short breaks on families with a disabled child: report one of the quantitative phase*. London: Department for Education, Ref: DFE-RR063.

Wescott, H L and Jones, D P H (1999) Annotation: The Abuse of Disabled Children. *Journal of Child Psychology and Psychiatry*, 40, pp 497–506.

Whitehurst, T (2006) Liberating silent voices – perspectives of children with profound and complex learning needs on inclusion. *British Journal of Learning Disabilities* vol 35, no1, pp 55–61.

Williams, P and Evans, M (2013) *Social Work with People with Learning Difficulties, Third Edition*, London: Learning Matters.

Wilson, K and Ryan, V (2005) *Play Therapy: A Non-Directive Approach for Children and Adolescents* (2nd edn). Elsevier: London.

Wing, L and Gould, J (1979). Severe impairments of social interaction and associated abnormalities in children: epidemiology and classification. *Journal of Autism & Developmental Disorders,* 9, pp 11–29. Available from the NAS Information Centre.

Websites

Autism Research Institute Sensory integration www.autism.com/symptoms_sensory_overview.

Contact a Family Research www.cafamily.org.uk/professionals/research/ (accessed 2 January 2016).

Department of Health (2014) The Care Act 2014 (c23) www.legislation.gov.uk/ukpga/2014/23/pdfs/ ukpga_20140023_en.pdf (accessed 27 April 2015).

Department of Health (2014) *Care and support statutory guidance: Issued under the Care Act 2014,* London: Department of Health. Available online www.gov.uk/government/uploads/system/uploads/ attachment_data/file/315993/Care-Act-Guidance.pdf (accessed 19 August 2015).

Department of Health (2014) *The Care Act and whole-family approaches,* London: Department of Health. Available online www.local.gov.uk/documents/10180/5756320/The+Care+Act+and+whole+family+appr oaches/080c323f-e653-4cea-832a-90947c9dc00c (accessed 19 August 2015).

Department of Health (2014) *Care and support statutory guidance: Issued under the Care Act 2014,* paragraphs 16.37–38, London: Department of Health. Available online www.gov.uk/government/uploads/system/uploads/attachment_data/file/315993/Care-Act-Guidance.pdf (accessed 19 August 2015).

DfES (2001) Special Educational Needs Code of Practice. Available online http://webarchive.national-archives.gov.uk/20130401151715/https://www.education.gov.uk/publications/eorderingdownload/ dfes%200581%20200mig2228.pdf (accessed 20 August 2015).

Dichter G S (2012) www.autismsciencefoundation.wordpress.com/2013/06/10/getting-a-picture-of-autism-what-weve-learned-from-neuroimaging-studies/ (accessed 29 September 2015).

HM Government Disability rights: employment www.gov.uk/rights-disabled-person/employment (accessed 9 August 2015).

HM Government Statutory Assessments under the Children Act 1989: Working together to safeguard children www.lscbchairs.org.uk/sitedata/files/working_together_2013.pdf (accessed 4 August 2015).

Laming, Lord (2003) The Victoria Climbié Inquiry: Report. Available online dera.ioe.ac.uk/6086/2/climbiereport.pdf (accessed 4 August 2015).

Moving on From Bowlby The assessment framework for children in need (2012) https://movingonfrom-bowlby.wordpress.com/tag/assessment-framework/ (accessed 21 October 2014).

My Aspergers Child 'Face-Blindness' in children and teens with Aspergers and high-functioning autism www.myaspergerschild.com/2012/03/face-blindness-in-children-and-teens.html (accessed 21 November 2015).

The National Archives The Disability Discrimination Act http://webarchive.nationalarchives.gov.uk/+/ www.dh.gov.uk/en/Publicationsandstatistics/Publications/PublicationsPolicyAndGuidance/Browsable/ DH_5855997 (accessed 5 October 2015).

The National Autistic Society Strategies and approaches www.autism.org.uk/approaches (accessed 10 November 2015).

The National Autistic Society Adult autism strategy www.autism.org.uk/en-gb/working-with/autism-strategy/the-autism-strategy-an-overview/adult-autism-strategy.aspx (accessed 10 November 2015).

NHS Autistic spectrum disorder www.nhs.uk/conditions/autistic-spectrum-disorder/Pages/Introduction. aspx (accessed 8 November 2015).

NHS Hearing tests for older babies and children www.nhs.uk/Conditions/Hearing-and-vision-tests-for-children/Pages/Introduction.aspx#children (accessed 13 September 2015).

Norburn, A (2013) Communicating effectively with children under five. Available online www.rip.org.uk/research-evidence/research-briefings/frontline/484-communicating-effectively-with-children-under-5 (accessed 16 November 2015).

Social Care Institute for Excellence Adult carer transition in practice under the Care Act 2014 (2015) www.scie.org.uk/care-act-2014/transition-from-childhood-to-adulthood/adult-carer-transition-in-practice/index.asp (accessed 20 October 2015).

Special educational needs code of practice www.gov.uk/government/uploads/system/uploads/attachment_data/file/273877/special_educational_needs_code_of_practice.pdf (accessed 6 August 2015).

Special educational needs and disability code of practice www.gov.uk/government/uploads/system/uploads/attachment_data/file/398815/SEND_Code_of_Practice_January_2015.pdf (accessed 6 August 2015).

Spurgeons www.spurgeons.org/ (accessed 14 February 2015).

UK Legislation The Children Act 1989 Section 22 5(C) www.legislation.gov.uk/ukpga/1989/41/section/22 (accessed 6 December 2015).

UK Legislation Chronically Sick and Disabled Persons Act (CSDPA) Chapter 44 www.legislation.gov.uk/ukpga/1970/44 [accessed 28 August 2015].

UK Legislation The Mental Capacity Act 2005 (C9) Part 1 – Persons who lack capacity www.legislation.gov.uk/ukpga/2005/9/contents (accessed 29 April 2015).

Autism and Asperger's syndrome What is ASD? www.asdcare.com/whatis.htm#triad.

Index